A Practical Guide to Cardiac Pacing

A Practical Guide to Cardiac Pacing

Fifth Edition

H. Weston Moses, M.D.
Clinical Associate Professor of Medicine, Southern Illinois University School of Medicine; Member, Prairie Cardiovascular Consultants, Ltd., Springfield, Illinois

Kriegh P. Moulton, M.D.
Clinical Assistant Professor of Medicine, Southern Illinois University School of Medicine; Director, Cardiac Electrophysiology, Prairie Cardiovascular Consultants, Ltd., Springfield, Illinois

Brian D. Miller, M.D.
Clinical Assistant Professor of Medicine, Southern Illinois University School of Medicine; Cardiac Electrophysiologist, Prairie Cardiovascular Consultants, Ltd., Springfield, Illinois

Joel A. Schneider, M.D.
Clinical Assistant Professor of Surgery, Southern Illinois University School of Medicine; Member, Prairie Cardiovascular Surgical Associates, Springfield, Illinois

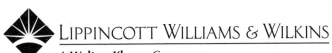

LIPPINCOTT WILLIAMS & WILKINS
A **Wolters Kluwer** Company
Philadelphia · Baltimore · New York · London
Buenos Aires · Hong Kong · Sydney · Tokyo

Acquisitions Editor: Ruth W. Weinberg
Developmental Editor: Alexandra T. Anderson
Production Editor: Rakesh Rampertab
Manufacturing Manager: Tim Reynolds
Cover Designer: Christine Jenny
Compositor: Lippincott Williams & Wilkins Desktop Division
Printer: Courier Westford

© 2000 by LIPPINCOTT WILLIAMS & WILKINS
227 East Washington Square
Philadelphia, PA 19106-3780 USA
LWW.com

Printed in the USA

Library of Congress Cataloging-in-Publication Data
A practical guide to cardiac pacing / H. Weston Moses . . . [et al.].—5th ed.
    p.; cm.
Includes bibliographical references and index.
ISBN 0-7817-1956-9
1. Cardiac pacing. I. Moses, H. Weston.
[DNLM: 1. Cardiac Pacing, Artifical. 2. Pacemaker, Artificial. WG 168 P895 2000]
RC684.P3 P75 2000
617.4′120645—dc21   99-046283

10 9 8 7 6 5 4 3 2 1

To our children:
Ann Moses, Wes Moses, and Amy Moses
Jennifer Bruse, Aaron Moulton, and Jason Moulton
Anthony Miller, Nicholas Miller, and Jordan Miller
M. Bret Schneider, Matthew Schneider, Roxanne Schneider,
and Cole Randle

Contents

Preface   ix

1. Indications for Pacing   1

2. Pacemaker Technology   27

3. Electrophysiology of Pacing   47

4. Programmability and Specialized Circuits   61

5. Types of Pacemakers and Hemodynamics of Pacing   75

6. Dual-chamber Pacing: Special Considerations   95

7. Rate-modulated Pacing   103

8. Implantable Cardioverter Defibrillator and Antitachycardia
    Pacing   111

9. Pacemaker Implantation   127

10. Follow-up of the Patient Who Has Received a Pacemaker   143

Glossary   167

Suggested Reading   181

Appendix I Conversion Chart   183

Appendix II Pacing Paradigms   185

Subject Index   197

Preface

A Practical Guide to Cardiac Pacing was written to acquaint the reader with basic pacing principles and terminology. In revising the text for its fifth edition, our goals were to emphasize the qualities that we believe have made the book successful in previous editions, while updating the text to keep pace with changes in technology and clinical advances. We have always viewed this book as a bridge between the beginner in pacing or general cardiologist and the engineers involved in designing pacemakers and electrophysiologists doing advanced pacemaker work. Every effort has been made to keep the text basic, and some discussions are deliberately simplified to serve as an appropriate framework for understanding pacemakers. As before, we have avoided naming specific pacemaker brands and models (a task more difficult than might be imagined).

The field of pacemakers is expanding so rapidly that a book this size cannot realistically be complete. We do, however, hope that emphasis on some of the basic principles, perhaps in an overly simplified manner will provide the basis for understanding evolving developments.

The role of private industry has been critical in developing the pacemaker and in educating clinicians about its use. Because of the complex characteristics of individual pacemakers, a text on cardiac pacing cannot hope to offer all the information needed to manage a pacemaker patient the way a pharmaceutical text can provide everything the clinician needs to know to manage a patient on a particular drug regimen. Still, we hope this book will provide a link between the standard areas of medical knowledge and areas of electrophysiology and technology not routinely encountered in medical education.

The authorship of the book has changed from past editions. Dr. George Taylor and Dr. James Dove, were previous authors, are acknowledged for their excellent work, much of which remains in this edition.

We are grateful for the perspective given by many individuals. Specifically, we thank Steven Allex, John Buysman, Ed Duffin, Steve Erickson, Lynne Hicks, Scott Iwen, Stella Kim, Stephen Mahle, Toby Markowitz, Terence Nadler, Jim Niebur, Diane Schuster, Wyatt Stahl, Lyn Stepaniak, and Steve Subera. We are also very grateful for help provided over the years by Serge Barold, Toshio Akiyama, and Paul Levine. We appreciate the secretarial assistance of Bridgett Wake and Beckie Hart. We are grateful for the artwork done since 1981 through the present by Don Biggerstaff, William Andrea, Gary Schnitz, John Sheedy, Thomas Broad, and Andra Ross. Our nurses, Theresa Thompson, Jane Scott, Karen Bade, and Trish Quintenz have been helpful with research.

Finally, the editorial assistance of Owsley Thunman of Springfield and Alexandra Anderson and Rakesh Rampertab of Lippincott Williams & Wilkins is greatly appreciated.

H.W.M.
K.P.M.
B.D.M.
J.A.S.

A Practical Guide to Cardiac Pacing

1

Indications for Pacing

INDICATIONS FOR PERMANENT PACEMAKER THERAPY

General Guidelines

The presence of symptoms remains the most compelling indication for pacemaker treatment. *Symptomatic bradycardia* is a term used to identify clinical manifestations associated with a heart rate that does not allow cardiac output to meet physiologic demands. Such symptoms include transient light-headedness, near-syncope or syncope, and symptoms suggestive of transient cerebral ischemia (e.g., light-headedness or atypical vertigo). In addition, more general symptoms of exercise intolerance and heart failure may be related to a slow heart rate. Patients exhibiting such symptoms attributable to a slow heart rate generally are candidates for cardiac pacing.

Patients with syncope or near-syncope usually have bradycardias that occur intermittently and therefore are not detected on the routine electrocardiogram (ECG). For such patients, ambulatory ECG monitoring (patient-activated event recordings, Holter monitoring, or inpatient telemetry) is essential to document the arrhythmia. Insertion of a pacemaker in a symptomatic patient who has not had documented arrhythmias may be followed by the embarrassing persistence of symptoms. Likewise, spontaneous termination of nonsustained atrial tachyarrhythmias can result in transient bradyarrhythmias and similar symptoms. These symptoms may be managed more appropriately by antiarrhythmic therapy aimed at suppressing the tachyarrhythmia. Only asymptomatic patients who have documented bradycardias that are associated with poor prognosis are candidates for pacemaker treatment.

An increasingly critical issue with pacemaker therapy is the high cost of cardiac pacing technology. Health care resources are finite, and pacemaker therapy is expensive. Because this area of medicine is easy to audit, intense scrutiny has become the rule. Third-party payers may deny reimbursement for nonindicated pacemakers. Unfortunately, the indication for permanent pacemaker treatment is not always clear-cut. In some cases, the clinician must deal with probabilities.

Sometimes patients will be treated with pacemakers in nebulous clinical situations, but this should occur only when clinical judgment indicates that the

1

potential benefit of a pacemaker outweighs its risks and expense. These issues represent the competing forces between minimizing health care costs and providing the best possible care for the individual patient. We believe the physician's primary obligation is to the patient, but this cannot, of course, be used as an excuse for careless clinical practice.

Atrioventricular Block

Nomenclature of Atrioventricular Block

It is important to note that the nomenclature of atrioventricular (AV) block refers to ECG patterns and not to pathophysiology of anatomic site of block, although these topics are the major theme of subsequent discussion.

First-degree AV block is defined as prolongation of the PR interval (onset of P wave to onset of QRS complex) beyond 0.20 seconds. With first-degree AV block, there is no true block but rather a "delay in AV conduction" longer than 0.20 seconds. Thus, no heartbeats are dropped. There is no evidence that patients with isolated first-degree AV block have reduced morbidity or mortality with permanent pacemaker placement, with the possible rare exception of pacing patients with congestive heart failure with a markedly long PR interval and *≈300 msec* improving the patients symptomatically with better atrial ventricular synchrony.

Second-degree AV block is characterized by intermittent failure of atrial depolarizations to reach the ventricle. There are two patterns of second-degree AV block. The first, type I, was described initially by Wenckebach in 1899 without use of ECG but based instead on observations of the waves of the jugular venous and carotid arterial pulse. Mobitz was able to describe the ECG manifestations of type I second-degree block in 1924 with demonstration of progressive prolongation of the PR interval in cycles preceding the dropped beat. This is alternatively referred to as the *Wenckebach phenomenon* or *Mobitz type I block*. The prognosis in patients with asymptomatic type I second-degree AV block tends to be good. The second pattern, or *Mobitz type II* second-degree block, refers to intermittent dropped beats preceded by constant PR intervals. Strictly speaking, Mobitz I and Mobitz II block refer to ECG patterns and not to anatomic location of the block. Because the AV node is most commonly the site of Mobitz I block and the infranodal tissue is most commonly the site of Mobitz II block, the ECG pattern is often equated with the anatomic location; however, unusual exceptions do exist.

Patients with second-degree AV block (either Mobitz type I or II) in whom every other beat is blocked have 2-to-1 block. It should be emphasized that 2-to-1 second-degree AV block is common and cannot be designated as either Mobitz I or Mobitz II. Those in whom only every third beat is conducted have 3-to-1 block. Those with two of three beats conducted, or every third beat blocked, have 3-to-2 block. Progression of Mobitz type II second-degree AV block to complete AV block is common, and the prognosis is improved with permanent pacemaker placement.

Third-degree AV block, also known as *complete AV block*, describes failure of any depolarizations to pass from the atria through the AV node to the ventricles. The atria beat regularly in response to the sinoatrial (SA) node. The ventricles beat independently in response to a pacemaker located in the proximal portion of the His bundle (junctional rhythm), often at a rate of 40 beats per minute (bpm) to 70 bpm. Alternatively, the subsidiary pacemaker site may be located within the distal Purkinje tissue with a rate less than 40 bpm. Patients with third-degree AV block who experience syncope have improved morbidity and mortality rates with permanent pacemaker implantation.

His Bundle Electrogram

Much of our understanding of the conduction anatomy of the heart has come from study of the intracardiac electrogram, often referred to as the *His bundle electrogram*. Depolarization of the AV node and the His bundle produces no deflection on the surface ECG; however, a closely spaced bipolar electrode can be positioned across the anterosuperior portion of the septal tricuspid valve leaflet, in close proximity to the His bundle. A depolarization spike originating from the common His bundle can be recorded (H spike, Fig. 1-1). On the intra-

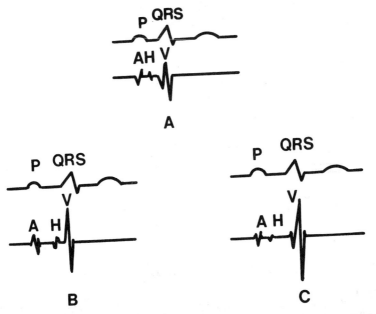

FIG. 1-1. His bundle recording. **A:** The normal His bundle recording demonstrates an A deflection corresponding to the P wave on the surface ECG. The H deflection occurs during the isoelectric period between the P wave and the QRS complex. The V deflection corresponds to the QRS complex. **B:** Prolonged AH interval (>140 msec) block within the AV node. **C:** Prolonged HV interval (>55 msec) block below the AV node.

cardiac ECG, atrial (A) depolarization precedes the H spike, and ventricular (V) depolarization follows the H spike. The interval between the atrial and His depolarizations (AH interval) reflects conduction through the AV node. The HV interval is the result of conduction in the bundle branch system between the His bundle and the ventricles. Thus, AH interval prolongation indicates a conduction abnormality within the AV node (above the His bundle); HV interval prolongation indicates an infranodal conduction abnormality. This technique for localizing conduction problems in the AV node or the infranodal conduction system has had a major impact on our understanding of AV block.

Pathophysiology of Atrioventricular Block

Atrioventricular Nodal Block

Impulse delay in the AV node may produce first-degree AV block, indicated by PR interval prolongation. Further deterioration of conduction within the AV node may result in second-degree block of the Wenckebach or Mobitz I variety (Fig. 1-2). To avoid confusion, subsequent discussion will refer only to

Location of heart block	Classification and ECG appearance	QRS duration	Origin of escape rhythm with complete heart block	Prognosis
AV Node block 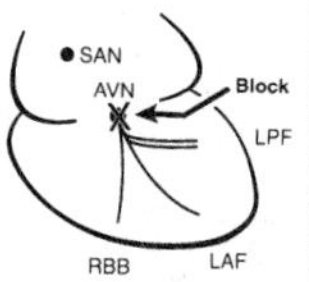	1. First degree AV block PR ≥ .22 sec. 2. Wenckebach, Mobitz I, block 3. Complete heart block	Normal (<0.12 sec.) (but may have associated bundle branch block	AVN usually heart rate ≥40 beats/min	Good
Infranodal block 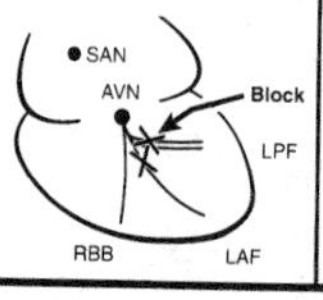	1. Mobitz II 2. Complete heart block	Wide (≥40 0.12 sec.)	Ventricular conduction system usually heart rate ≤20 beats/min.	Poor

FIG. 1-2. Nodal versus infranodal heart block. A statistically and clinically significant association between ECG pattern and the anatomic location of block is shown. In general, block within the AV node has a good prognosis (with some exceptions), and block of second or third degree below the AV node has a poor prognosis. The unusual situation of Mobitz I second-degree AV block in association with a wide QRS complex is not depicted in the figure. This type of block can be caused by nodal or infranodal block and may require investigation with electrophysiologic studies. (SAN, sinoatrial node; AVN, atrioventricular node; RBB, right bundle branch; LPF, left posterior fascicle; LAF, left anterior fascicle.)

Mobitz I block and not to Wenckebach block. *Mobitz I block* is characterized by lengthening of the PR interval in sequential beats until there is a nonconducted P wave. The simplest way to distinguish between Mobitz I and Mobitz II is to look for a difference in the PR interval in the beats *preceding* and *following* the dropped beat. If a difference between these two PR intervals is greater than 0.02 seconds, then Mobitz I is present. If the difference is less than 0.02 seconds, then Mobitz II is present. Often, Mobitz I may progress to a higher grade of second-degree AV block known as 2-to-1 AV block, in which alternate P waves are not conducted. Although this is most commonly associated with Mobitz I, it should be termed *2-to-1 AV block* because a distinction cannot be made between Mobitz I and Mobitz II. A long rhythm strip usually catches periods of less than 2-to-1 block and can clarify whether Mobitz I or Mobitz II is present.

Because both first-degree AV block and Mobitz I second-degree block most commonly result from block within the AV node, and not the infranodal conduction system, the QRS duration is usually normal. A wide QRS complex in a setting of Mobitz I block would indicate block within the AV node and coexisting bundle branch block, but a remote chance exists of Mobitz I block occurring in an infranodal structure. Although Mobitz II is far less common than Mobitz I, a wide QRS complex nearly always is associated with the former. A common misinterpretation of Mobitz II occurs in the condition known as *vagotonia*, in which there may be no difference in the PR intervals before and after the blocked beat. There is always a lengthening of the PP interval (sinus slowing), however, which occurs concomitant with the transient AV block and is seen frequently in anyone with enhanced vagal tone, commonly observed at nighttime during sleep.

Mobitz I second-degree block may progress to third-degree block, although it does so less commonly than Mobitz II block. When third-degree AV block occurs at the level of the AV node, the takeover pacemaker is located high in the conduction system, usually in the common bundle of His. Pacemakers this high in the infranodal conduction system usually have an intrinsic rate of 40 to 70 bpm. The rare condition of congenital complete AV block is most often of AV junctional origin. Such patients with complete AV block usually have a junctional rhythm and narrow QRS complexes. Their heart rates increase with exercise, and pacemaker therapy may not be needed.

Mobitz I second-degree block can be found as a normal occurrence in young people, particularly in well-trained athletes. Certain antiarrhythmic drugs such as class II, class IV, and digitalis glycosides also can cause Mobitz I AV block. These patients are usually asymptomatic, and pacemaker therapy usually is not indicated. On rare occasions, however, elderly patients have severe degenerative disease in the conduction system, and Mobitz type I block leads to symptomatic bradycardias requiring pacemaker therapy.

The His bundle electrogram in patients with block within the AV node shows prolongation of the AH interval with a normal HV interval (see Fig. 1-1).

Infranodal Atrioventricular Block

Block below the AV node (see Fig. 1-2) involves the bundle of His or the three fascicles arising from the bundle of His. The PR interval may be normal. In contrast with AV nodal block, the PR interval does not differ when comparing the cardiac cycles preceding or following the blocked beat. Mobitz II block almost always is associated with bundle branch block and broad QRS complexes.

Patients with Mobitz II block frequently progress to third-degree (complete) AV block, and the risk of sudden death is high in this group of patients. Therefore, Mobitz II AV block is an indication for pacemaker therapy regardless of symptoms. The His bundle electrogram in patients with block below the AV node shows prolongation of the HV interval.

Complete Atrioventricular Block

Complete AV block indicates total interruption of conduction of impulses from the atria to the ventricles. As a result, there is a lack of any fixed relationship between P waves and QRS complexes. Block can develop at any level in the conduction system. Block in the AV node usually is associated with narrow QRS complexes and a subsidiary pacemaker with a rate of 40 to 70 bpm. This pacemaker often responds to stimulation of the autonomic nervous system. For example, a patient with block within the AV node and a resting heart rate of 40 bpm may have an increase in heart rate with exercise.

Complete AV block due to interruption of infranodal conduction usually is associated with a wide QRS complex and a slow takeover pacemaker. Many patients with complete block below the AV node have heart rates of less than 40 bpm. Most cases of complete AV block encountered clinically are infranodal, especially in elderly patients, who constitute the majority of patients requiring pacemaker therapy. Many of these patients do not have clinically apparent heart disease. Rather, the pathophysiology of AV block in many elderly patients is a fibrotic, degenerative process involving the conduction system below the AV node known as *Lev's* or *Lenegre's disease*.

Permanent Pacemaker Therapy in Atrioventricular Block

Third-Degree Atrioventricular Block

With third-degree AV block, there is dissociation of atrial and ventricular rhythm. Most patients have block below the AV node and are symptomatic. The survival rate for symptomatic patients is improved with pacemaker therapy. The occasional patient who is asymptomatic with third-degree AV block, especially if the ventricular rate is less than 40 bpm, usually becomes symptomatic, is at risk for sudden death, and should be paced. Occasionally, patients with complete AV block and bradycardia are unaware of having a mental or physical deficit until the pacemaker has been inserted. The rare asymptomatic patient with complete AV block in the AV node may not require pacing.

Mobitz II Second-Degree Atrioventricular Block

Most patients with Mobitz II block have symptomatic bradycardia, and the indication for pacemaker therapy is clear. Those with symptoms (the majority) are at high risk for developing complete AV block and Stokes–Adams attacks, usually within a few months. Asymptomatic Mobitz II second-degree AV block has been categorized as an equivocal indication for pacemaker treatment. If not paced, such patients should be monitored carefully for the appearance of symptoms or progression of heart block. Ambulatory monitoring using an event recorder to exclude severe intermittent bradycardia may be useful. Unless symptoms occur more often than once daily, 24-hour Holter monitoring is not likely to disclose symptomatic periods of bradyarrhythmia but may uncover asymptomatic periods of Mobitz II AV block. True asymptomatic Mobitz II block is rare, and we generally recommend pacemaker therapy.

Mobitz I Second-Degree Atrioventricular Block

Usually patients with Mobitz I second-degree AV block are asymptomatic and not at risk for symptoms or sudden death. Occasionally, however, patients with heart block localized to the AV node are symptomatic, and pacemaker therapy is required. Ambulatory monitoring is necessary to demonstrate or disprove an association of bradycardia and symptoms. For such patients, negatively dromotropic drugs (e.g., digitalis, beta-adrenergic blockers, verapamil) may produce Mobitz I block. Thus, the medication should be discontinued if at all possible and the patient observed by inpatient ambulatory monitoring for continued manifestations of AV block before committing to permanent pacemaker implantation.

High-Risk Bundle Branch Block

Chronic right or left bundle branch block are not indications for pacemaker therapy. The long-term stability of AV conduction in combination right bundle branch block (RBBB) and left anterior fascicular block (LAFB) has been questioned. This pattern of infranodal block is seen commonly because of the anatomic proximity of the right bundle and left anterior fascicle in the interventricular septum. Prospective observation of patients with RBBB and LAFB has shown an insignificant increase in risk for developing complete AV block. Although patients with bifascicular or chronic BBB have increased cardiovascular mortality, conduction abnormalities and bradycardias are not the cause of death in a sufficient number of patients to warrant prophylactic pacing. Sudden death may be the result of ventricular arrhythmias because many of these patients have coronary artery disease, left ventricular dysfunction, or both. The indication for permanent pacemaker therapy with bifascicular block is the documentation of bradycardias in association with symptoms.

There was hope that invasive electrophysiologic studies would identify patients with infranodal conduction abnormalities who were at high risk for progression to complete AV block. As noted earlier, the His bundle electrogram has been invaluable in identifying sites of block in a variety of clinical settings. Prolongation of the AH interval indicates block in the AV node, and HV interval prolongation indicates block below the AV node. With bifascicular block, only one of the three fascicles remains. A long HV interval in such a patient with bifascicular block invariably identifies a conduction abnormality in the third fascicle. It seems reasonable to assume that this subset of patients with bifascicular block and long HV intervals would be at greatest risk for developing complete AV block. Experience has not demonstrated that measurement of HV interval reliably distinguishes high-risk from low-risk patients, however, and thus the clinical utility of the intracardiac electrogram is not proved in patients with bifascicular block. Although pacing had been suggested for those with BBB and long HV intervals, prospective studies did not substantiate this approach. His bundle studies in asymptomatic patients with bifascicular block are usually not necessary; however, HV interval prolongation in symptomatic patients with BBB may identify which patients are likely to develop complete heart block.

An additional maneuver suggested for identifying the high-risk patient with bifascicular block is rapid atrial pacing. Patients who are susceptible to developing Mobitz II or complete AV block may do so when the conduction system is stressed by pacing at rapid rates.

The His bundle electrogram may prove useful in other clinical situations. Occasionally, patients with Mobitz I block have associated BBB, and demonstration of a prolonged AH interval but normal HV interval indicates that the block is located in the AV node. Mobitz I block, which occurs rarely in the His bundle below the AV node, may be diagnosed by prolongation of the HV interval and is an indication for pacemaker therapy. Rarely, patients with Mobitz II block have narrow QRS complexes diagnosed by prolonged HV intervals (intrahisian block).

Finally, there are limits as to how strict clinicians can be when making a decision about the individual patient. Over the last decade, the reliability of pacemakers has steadily improved, and pacing generators have become progressively smaller, reducing the morbidity and discomfort associated with pacemaker therapy. The use of invasive cardiac electrophysiologic studies and equivocal noninvasive studies in patients with symptoms has benefitted some patients in helping to determine the etiology of their symptoms. For example, it must be remembered that the syncope in a patient with a history of anterior wall myocardial infarction (MI) and bifascicular block is commonly secondary to ventricular tachycardia rather than to heart block, and therefore empirically implanting a pacemaker is potentially beneficial for the heart block but will not solve the problem or prevent morbidity and mortality.

Sick Sinus Syndrome

The sick sinus syndrome is the condition most commonly treated by pacemaker placements. This disorder includes a variety of cardiac arrhythmias, all characterized by SA arrest or SA exit block. The result of both is sinus brady-cardia. The junctional escape mechanism may be inappropriately slow in patients with sick sinus syndrome.

Patients with SA node dysfunction often have alternating supraventricular tachycardias and bradycardias. This seemingly paradoxical juxtaposition of rapid and slow heart rhythms has resulted in the term *tachy-brady syndrome*. Such alterations in rhythm often come about because of the spontaneous termi-nation of a primary atrial tachyarrhythmia. On abrupt cessation of the exces-sively rapid stimulation of the sinus node, fatigue of this pacemaker site becomes manifest as a transient bradyarrhythmia. This phenomenon, referred to as *overdrive suppression* of the sinus node, is markedly exaggerated in patients with the sick sinus syndrome. Supraventricular tachycardias include ectopic atrial tachycardia, AV nodal reentry, atrioventricular reentry, and paroxysmal atrial fibrillation or flutter. A patient may experience a variety of these arrhyth-mias, moving from one form of supraventricular tachycardia to another within a fairly short time. Bouts of tachycardia often are followed by disturbingly long SA pauses with associated symptoms of reduced cerebral blood. Failure to appreciate the likelihood of SA node dysfunction in this situation may be disas-trous. Cardioversion of slow atrial fibrillation may be complicated by asystole or profound sinus bradycardia. Patients with disorders of the SA node may have concomitant AV node dysfunction as well.

Although the sick sinus syndrome can occur in young people, it is most com-mon in patients aged older than 60 years. Patients usually present with dizziness or syncope but may have vague and nonspecific complaints. Diagnosis depends on demonstrating arrhythmias at the time that symptoms occur, which can be accomplished by using the event recorder as a form of ambulatory monitoring. The event recorder is commonly given to the patient for a duration of 2 to 4 weeks (or however long it takes to document symptoms). Holter monitoring is effective only when symptoms occur more frequently than once daily because it is a 24-hour recording device. Thus, the choice of the ambulatory monitoring device depends on symptom frequency.

Profound bradycardia with associated symptoms is an obvious indication for pacemaker therapy when culpable medications have been excluded. Occasion-ally, patients with less severe bradycardia who have long sinus pauses without obvious symptoms also may need pacemakers. Clinical judgment is required in this situation, and the decision to recommend a pacemaker is at times arbitrary.

An additional use for pacemaker therapy in patients with sick sinus syndrome is support of heart rate when pharmacologic blockade of tachycardias results in symptomatic bradycardia. For example, some patients with paroxysmal atrial fibrillation may require doses of beta-adrenergic blockers or digoxin that cause an unacceptable level of bradycardia. Pacing is needed so that these patients can tolerate their other antiarrhythmic therapy.

Invasive electrophysiologic studies have proved relatively useless in evalua-tion of the sick sinus syndrome. The SA node recovery time, measured by abrupt cessation of rapid atrial pacing, usually is abnormal in patients with the sick sinus syndrome. In patients with clear-cut sick sinus syndrome, there is little need for this study. Furthermore, in many patients with syncope from other causes, sinus node recovery time may be abnormal and thus unrelated to the cause of syncope. For those with probable sick sinus syndrome in whom the diagnosis cannot be established by history and ambulatory monitoring, SA node recovery time lacks sensitivity and specificity. A measure of conduction between SA node and atrium, called the *SA conduction time,* also lacks sensitivity and specificity. Ambulatory monitoring remains the most useful diagnostic tool. In some difficult situations, however, a combination of SA node function tests, electrophysiologic tests to induce tachycardia, and ambulatory monitoring may help provide a diagnosis.

Myocardial Infarction

Permanent pacemaker therapy after MI is required relatively infrequently. Indications are related to the extent of damage to the conduction system. The requirement for temporary pacing in an acute MI does not necessarily mean permanent pacing is indicated. Inferior and posterior wall MIs are associated with significant transient bradycardias and AV block conditions that often are linked to the stimulation of ventricular C-fiber receptors. These receptors are involved with enhanced vagal tone and are seen with the Bezold–Jarisch reflex, which can last for a week or more, but are usually temporary and therefore rarely require permanent pacing. Some patients with an anterior wall MI and significant transient disruption of the infranodal conduction system may be at risk for sudden death, however, and permanent pacing is indicated in this situation. Table 1-1

TABLE 1–1. *Indications for permanent cardiac pacemakers*

I. Indications for permanent pacing in acquired atrioventricular (nodal or infranodal) block in adults
  A. Pacing recommended or reasonable
    1. Third-degree AV block, either nodal or infranodal, associated with bradycardia that is symptomatic
    2. Third-degree nodal AV block that results in periods of asystole of over 3 sec or heart rate <40 bpm, even if asymptomatic
    3. Third-degree infranodal AV block, or second-degree infranodal block Mobitz II, even without symptoms or significant pauses
    4. Intermittent third-degree AV block, especially if infranodal, probably if nodal, depending on the clinical circumstances
    5. After catheter ablation of the AV junction, done for atrial fibrillation with an uncontrolled rapid ventricular response (an adnunctive ventricular pacemaker is required)
    6. Postoperative AV block that does not resolve "shortly" (usually within 2 days) after surgery
    7. Symptomatic second-degree AV block regardless whether it is nodal or infranodal
    8. Incidental finding at electrophysiologic study of a markedly prolonged HV internal (≥ 100 msec) in asymptomatic individuals; also, an incidental finding at electrophysiologic study of pacing-induced infra-HIS block that is not physiologic
    9. A less clear-cut problem is first-degree AV block with left ventricular dysfunction with symptoms that appear to be relieved by shortening the PR interval with a dual-chamber pacemaker (we have not used this indication)

TABLE 1–1. *Continued.*

B. Pacing not recommended
    1. First-degree AV block, asymptomatic Mobitz I second-degree AV block (assuming it is not due to block in the HIS or infra-His area), transient AV block likely to resolve, for example, due to drug toxicity or Lyme disease
    2. It is generally recognized that bifascicular block without symptoms (with or without first-degree AV block) does not require pacing

II. Indications for permanent pacemaker after the acute phase of myocardial infarction
  A. Pacing recommended or reasonable
    1. Third-degree AV block or persistent Mobitz II second-degree block after an anterior wall myocardial infarction
    2. Transient Mobitz second-degree or third-degree infranodal block associated with bundle branch block, after an anterior wall MI
  B. Pacing not recommended
    AV block due to an inferior wall MI occurs within the AV node and both Mobitz I second-degree and third-degree AV block will almost always resolve without the need for a pacemaker

III. Indications for permanent pacing in sinus node dysfunction
  A. Pacing recommended or reasonable
    1. Sinus node dysfunction with bradycardia leading to symptoms would include bradycardia due to required long-term drug therapies
    2. Symptomatic chronically slow heart rate
    3. Symptomatic bradycardia–tachycardia syndrome, especially if medication to treat the tachyarrhythmia will aggravate the bradyarrhythmia
  B. Pacing not recommended
    1. Asymptomatic sinus node dysfunction (sometimes with Mobitz I second-degree AV block) including athletic persons with high vagal tone

IV. Pacing indications to prevent tachycardia
  A. Pacing recommended or reasonable
    1 Sustained pause-dependent ventricular tachycardia with or without prolonged QT interval (electrophysiologic often recommended)
    2. Some high-risk patients with congenital long QT syndrome (electrophysiology opinion recommended)
  B. Pacing not recommended
    1. Suppression of ventricular tachycardia not well documented to be pause dependent

V. Indications for permanent pacemakers that automatically detect and pace to terminate tachyarrhythmias
  Some work has been done with supraventricular tachycardias reproducibly terminated by tachy-pacing in a specialized area of electrophysiology
  The automatic implantable cardioverter defibrillator systems generally now have tachy-pacing as part of the system to attempt to terminate ventricular tachycardia with pacing before attempting a shock

VI. Indications for permanent pacing in hypersensitive carotid sinus syndrome accompanied by syncope or neurocardiogenic syncope
  Recurrent syncope caused by tilt table testing of carotid sinus stimulation documented on study and with a significant bradycardiac component, not just a vasodepressor component (we have found this an uncommon indication)

VII. Indications for permanent pacing in children and adolescents
  This specialized area is best addressed by a pediatric cardiologist/electrophysiologist; however, AV block or sinus-node dysfunction can occur in congenital heart disease or in relation to surgery for congenital heart disease; long-term QT syndrome can occur in the pediatric population

VIII. Pacing indication for hypertrophic cardiomyopathy
  Some studies indicate that dual-chamber pacing with a short AV interval and stimulation at the RV apex will improve symptoms in patients with idiopathic hypertrophic cardiomyopathy

IX. Indications for pacing for dilated cardiomyopathy
  Some studies indicate that pacing of a patient with dilated cardiomyopathy for optimal PR interval and possibly dual-site pacing in the left ventricle for more synchronous LV contraction will improve symptoms. The use is investigational

X. Indications for pacing to prevent atrial fibrillation
  Some studies indicate that atrial pacing may reduce episodes of recurrent atrial fibrillation (some studies use two atrial sites to pace); This not an established procedure

AV = atrioventricular; MI = myocardial infarction; RV, right ventricle.

outlines recommendations for permanent pacing after MI, but these should be considered only rough guidelines.

Hypersensitive Carotid Sinus Syndrome

There are three types of carotid sinus hypersensitivity:

1. *Cardioinhibitor reflex* results from an increased parasympathetic tone and a decreased sympathetic tone as a response to carotid sinus stimulation or manipulation. Such stimulation may result in a fall in sinus note rate, prolongation of the PR interval with a prolonged conduction through the AV node, and a consequent drop in heart rate and blood pressure.

2. *Vasodepressor carotid hypertension* is due to reduction in sympathetic tone resulting in a loss of peripheral vascular resistance. There may or may not be an associated change in heart rate. Often, the heart rate may increase by reflex response to the lowered peripheral vascular resistance.

3. *Mixed vasodepressor* and *cardioinhibitory forms*: Both decreased heart rate and lowered peripheral vascular resistance may contribute to hypotension. Usually, the effect on heart rate is brief and transient. The effect on peripheral vascular resistance usually outlasts the slowing of heart rate by a significant time. As a person ages, the hypersensitive carotid sinus reflex becomes more common, but it is not necessarily related to any symptoms. If a patient is found to have a carotid sinus hypersensitivity and syncope, other etiologies of the syncope must be ruled out before assuming that this augmented reflex apparently has caused the patient's symptoms.

If a patient has a pure cardioinhibitory form of carotid sinus syndrome (rare), a resultant ventricular backup pacing to help support the patient's heart rate during the times of carotid sinus stimulation is helpful in prevention of the patient's symptoms. If, however, a patient has a pure vasodepressor hypersensitivity, the use of a pacemaker is of no benefit. If a patient has a mixed cardioinhibitory and vasodepressor reflex, the use of the ventricular pacing may be somewhat beneficial. The use of backup AV sequential pacing could prove to be even more beneficial; however, it may not resolve a patient's total symptoms but only blunt their effects (see Table 1-1). A form of pacing with hysteresis may be potentially useful. With sudden slowing of the heart rate, as occurs in the vasovagal reaction, the heart is paced rapidly for a brief time in an effort to maintain a reasonable blood pressure and cardiac output.

Hypertrophic Obstructive Cardiomyopathy

Hypertrophic obstructive cardiomyopathy (HOCM) is a familial cardiomyopathy in which the left ventricular wall is asymmetrically thickened. The interventricular septum thickness significantly exceeds that of the opposing posterolateral wall. The hemodynamics of HOCM are those of subvalvular aortic stenosis, in which a pressure gradient exists across the left ventricular outflow tract. During ventricular contraction, a progressive degree of outflow tract obstruction results in both impaired cardiac output (dynamic outflow tract obstruction) and various degrees of mitral regurgitation caused by the inappropriate systolic anterior motion (SAM) of the anterior mitral leaflet. By altering the sequence of activation of the ventricles, the ventricular contractile pattern can be changed in a way to lessen the degree of outflow tract obstruction. The conventional site of ventricular pacing is within the right ventricular apex, and pacing from this site can favorably alter the degree of obstruction. To prevent ventricular activation from proceeding over the normal AV conduction system, the DDD (or dual chamber) pacemaker used must use a fairly short AV interval (<150 msec). In this way, "pure" right ventricular apical pacing is guaranteed. Whereas this approach to treating HOCM remains a possible indication for permanent pacing, it should be reserved for patients in whom attempts at medical therapy have failed.

SYNCOPE SUMMARIZED

We have discussed the indications for a pacemaker, but the clinician is often presented with a patient experiencing syncope [loss of consciousness (LOC)] and then must decide whether pacemaker placement is appropriate. We therefore present a brief review of syncope, including noncardiac causes.

Syncope remains a relatively common problem. It is experienced by at least 20% of all adults by age 75, causes about 3% of all emergency room visits, and accounts for 1% to 2% of all hospitalizations.

Syncope can be caused by a primary electric disturbance of the brain (seizure) or by a marked reduction in cerebral perfusion pressure, leading to a global brain problem. *Regional* reductions in cerebral blood flow (e.g., embolic phenomena) do not cause syncope unless the reticular activating system is the target, in which case results are often catastrophic and the patient may not awaken. Although the electroencephalogram (EEG) occasionally may disclose a seizure focus, carotid ultrasound testing is uninformative in the workup of syncope. Vertebrobasilar syndrome is an inferred cause only in rare cases where both carotids are occluded and usually is accompanied by a history of gait disturbance. A common metabolic cause of syncope is hypoglycemia, and so a quick fingerstick can be helpful. Because of its significant cost, electrophysiologic testing should be reserved for patients with a high-risk profile in whom head-up tilt testing is negative (see below).

Syncope is classified into two categories: *cardiovascular* and *noncardiovascular*. This distinction is important because cardiovascular causes have a 20% to 25% 2-year mortality and therefore must be ruled out, whereas noncardiovascular causes have only a 2% to 4% 2-year mortality.

I. Cardiovascular causes of syncope
   A. Cardiac arrhythmias (usually ventricular tachyarrhythmias, less often bradyarrhythmias)
   B. Aortic stenosis
   C. Hypertropic obstructive cardiomyopathy
   D. Pulmonary embolism
   E. Aortic dissection
   F. Pulmonary hypertension
II. Noncardiovascular causes of syncope
   A. Neurogenic syncope
      1. Vasovagal syncope
      2. Vasodepressor syncope
      3. Autonomic dysfunction (diabetes and old age)
   B. Seizure disorders
   C. Orthostatic hypotension
      1. Drug-induced
      2. Idiopathic (Shy–Drager and Bradbury–Eggleston)
   D. Carotid sinus hypersensitivity
   E. Acute hypoglycemia

The three most common causes are ventricular tachyarrhythmias, neurogenic syncope, and seizure disorders. In addition, medications often cause or contribute to syncope.

The differential diagnosis also may include vertigo, in which the history shows the typical "spinning room" sensation exacerbated by head movement and rarely includes LOC.

Diagnostic Clues

Frequently, physical injury associated with syncope suggests the presence of a ventricular tachyarrhythmia. Injury occurs because the patient has little warning that LOC is imminent.

With ventricular tachycardia, palpitation is not always present, and chest pain (due to the tachycardia, not ischemia) can be an associated manifestation. The patient with a history of coronary artery disease, particularly a prior MI, who exhibits episodic dizziness lasting for brief periods should be referred for electrophysiologic evaluation.

Often, patients with serious cardiac arrhythmias and syncope also have seizure-like involuntary movements during the arrhythmia. These movements may be misinterpreted as grand mal seizures because incontinence can occur with them. Postictal states do not follow a prolonged nonsustained arrhythmia, however, and seizures do not require cardiopulmonary resuscitation (CPR) and defibrillation. Often, the sequence of events can be tricky: Patients with neurogenic syncope may not have a discernible pulse because of the low rate and pressure. In such cases, CPR may have been done to "revive" these patients.

Neurogenic syncope usually is heralded by a prodrome that may include nausea, weakness, pallor, a "sinking feeling," pressure in the epigastrium, diaphoresis, and a feeling of warmth. Yawning and sleepiness are not uncommon. Neurogenic syncope often is associated with specific circumstances (situational syncope), such as micturition, defecation, cough, or abrupt pain from a visceral or cutaneous site. Painful or emotional experiences, hot and humid weather conditions, relative dehydration, and a recent history of strenuous exertion are all potential precipitating factors. Patients tend to be in the younger age group (vasovagal) but can be older. Autonomic dysfunction usually is seen in patients aged over 65 years. Patients with presyncope usually note that their symptoms diminish when they lie down.

Head-up tilt testing (HUTT) is commonly used to diagnose neurogenic syncope and to identify which type is present. The procedure usually is carried out in the catheterization laboratory with the patient secured to a table capable of tilting to 80 degrees while intraartial pressure is monitored continuously (Fig. 1-3). The duration of the test is usually 20 minutes. Vasovagal syncope is diagnosed when a precipitous fall in blood pressure is accompanied by a reduction in heart rate (low 40s or lower). *Vasodepressor syncope* is hypotension not associated with decreased heart rate. Autonomic dysfunction is diagnosed by a gradual (not precipitous) fall in blood pressure without any significant change in heart rate. It eventually reaches levels associated with LOC. Patients with autonomic dysfunction also demonstrate an abnormal response to the Valsalva

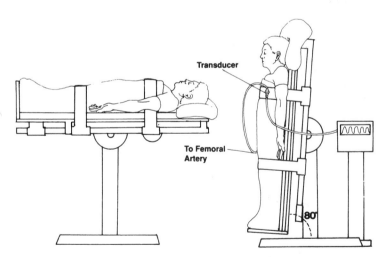

FIG. 1-3. Head-up tilt test. The patient is secured to the table in the horizontal position with straps over the chest and knee areas. A foot board should be in place and positioned securely at the bottom of the feet. Intra-arterial pressure monitoring is desirable. One must always remember to tape the transducer against the left chest wall at the level of the phlebostatic axis so that when the patient is brought to the upright position, there will be no change in the orientation of the transducer to the heart.

maneuver in that they do not exhibit blood pressure overshoot when the maneuver is terminated.

During HUTT, it is essential to perform carotid sinus massage (CSM) to uncover any carotid sinus hypersensitivity. There are pronounced differences in blood pressure responses to CSM when the patient is upright compared with when the patient is supine. Reproduction of clinical symptoms is important because some patients may have "hyperactive" carotid sinuses but do not faint.

It is best to measure intraarterial pressure with an indwelling catheter during HUTT. The use of an arm cuff may lead to inaccurate pressure readings and also may fail to warn of a precipitous drop in pressure. Another benefit of direct pressure measurements is the ability to diagnose pseudohypertension. In this situation, the wall of the larger arteries (brachial) is stiff and requires cuff pressures much greater than the actual systolic blood pressure to collapse the artery and to permit auscultation of the Korotkoff's sounds. Intraarterial pressure may be 150, but the cuff would indicate 190. Thus, the patient may be receiving therapy for hypertension when it is not truly present. The antihypertensive medications may reduce the patient's upright pressure to the 90s and set the stage for syncope.

The following medications commonly contribute to syncope: antihypertensives (all of them), tricyclic antidepressants, phenothiazine, and quinidine/quinine, to name a few. A common clinical situation is that of the elderly patient with a touch of autonomic dysfunction, a history of hypertension, and deficient fluid intake. This patient is on a diuretic and any one of the step II drugs. Under such circumstances, it is useful to withdraw the medications and establish a diagnosis of hypertension by having the patient take blood pressure measurements twice a day, once in the early morning and again during some active period of the day. Measurements are made for a minimum of 2 weeks and reported. Three or more systolic readings greater than 190 and diastolic greater than 100 should be reported. If, at the end of this testing period, the readings are acceptable, the drugs need not be resumed, and the syncope problem should cease. If hypertension does exist, monotherapy (using a beta-adrenergic blocker first) with careful blood pressure monitoring is indicated.

Treatment

The following is a list of treatment approaches for neurogenic syncope:

1. Withdraw potentially offending medications. Review the list of unusual diseases: Addison's, pyridoxine deficiency, pernicious anemia, multiple sclerosis, Shy–Drager, Bradbury–Eggleston, and tabes dorsalis. Alcoholism and diabetes mellitus are common in patients with syncope.

2. Encourage increased salt intake (this is not possible for the patient with a history of hypertension or heart failure). If increased salt intake is not possible, recommend nonprescription salt tablets (one or two tablets taken orally twice daily) and reassess in 2 weeks. Mild edema may occur in a small number of

patients. If this approach is not successful, medodrine, 5–10 mg potid taken orally two or three times daily, may be added.

3. Consider alternative drugs:
    a. Beta-adrenergic blockers
    b. Disopyramide, sustained-release tablets, 150 mg orally three times daily
    c. Scopolamine patch, one topically every third day

4. Try nonpharmacologic approaches, such as thigh-high support stockings and avoidance of prolonged immobility. Because the patient usually knows when an attack is imminent, he or she should be advised to lie flat on his or her back immediately, no matter the location.

5. It may be advisable to restrict driving for as long as 6 months if necessary or until there is a clear-cut response to therapy.

6. Refer the patient if palpitation-associated syncope occurs or if the patient has a history of significantly impaired left ventricular function. Referral is always advisable when the clinician is uncomfortable with the situation or when the suggested methods of treatment have not been successful.

INDICATIONS FOR TEMPORARY PACEMAKER THERAPY

Atrioventricular Block with Myocardial Infarction

The approach to patients with inferior MI is quite different from the approach to patients with anterior MI and is based on the pathophysiology of AV block caused by acute ischemia.

Inferior Myocardial Infarction

Inferior MI follows occlusion of the artery supplying the inferior wall of the left ventricle (Fig. 1-4), usually the right coronary artery, and also is the origin of the artery to the AV node. AV block with inferior MI therefore follows ischemia of the AV node. As in other forms of AV nodal block, it is characterized by a Mobitz I pattern (see Fig. 1-2). AV nodal block in the early stages of infarction may be aggravated by the increase in vagal tone that is common with inferior MI. Complete AV block may occur, but it is associated with a subsidiary pacemaker with a fairly rapid intrinsic rate that is high in the His–Purkinje system. This bradycardia usually responds to atropine or theophylline therapy. QRS complexes are narrow, as is usually the case with AV nodal block (unless coincidental BBB is present). Collateral blood flow to the AV node is good, and a return of normal function is the rule. Even with complete heart block, prognosis is good because heart block tends to be transient.

Temporary pacing is needed infrequently in patients with inferior MI and AV block. Temporary pacemaker therapy is necessary when (a) there is persistent and symptomatic bradycardia unresponsive to drug therapy, (b) ventricular irritability is aggravated by bradycardia, or (c) the patient has pump failure as a

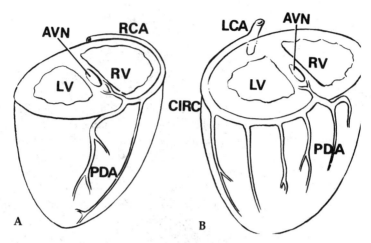

FIG. 1-4. AV nodal block in inferior wall MI. **A:** A dominant right coronary artery with an AV nodal artery coming off the right coronary artery. The patent ductus arteriosus (PDA) is running down the posterior portion of the heart (heart is shown from the back). **B:** An inferior wall myocardial infarction (MI) caused by occlusion of a dominant circumflex. In this case the AV nodal artery comes off the dominant circumflex, as does the posterior descending artery (again you are viewing the heart from the back). The actual cause of AV nodal block in this situation may be somewhat more complex than is described and may involve vasovagal effects or other neurogenic factors independent of pure AV node ischemia. (Modified from original artwork by Dr. Toshio Akiyama.)

result of bradycardia. Generally, a return to normal AV conduction occurs within a few days of acute inferior MI, but some patients have abnormal AV conduction for longer periods. The indication for permanent pacemaker therapy in acute inferior MI is persistent, symptomatic bradycardia, which is rare. Transient heart block noted in the early phase of an acute inferior MI, without symptoms and with a reasonable escape rate, is not an indication for temporary or permanent pacing.

Anterior Myocardial Infarction

In patients with acute anterior MI, AV block is usually a more serious matter than that with inferior MI. Blood flow to the AV node is intact, and AV block is a result of necrosis of the interventricular septum and the infranodal conduction system (Fig. 1-5). Selective block of portions of the infranodal conduction system often precedes complete AV block and should be considered a warning signal.

Patients with anterior MI and infranodal conduction abnormalities may develop complete AV block precipitously and with disastrous clinical consequences. Placement of a prophylactic pacemaker has clear advantages over efforts to a place a pacemaker during resuscitation in cases of cardiac arrest. On

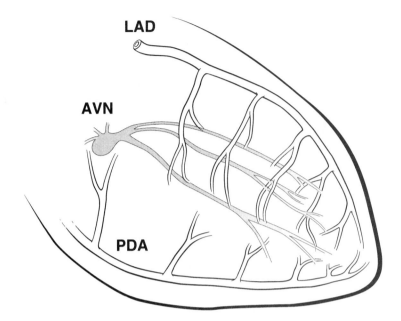

FIG. 1-5. Infranodal block in anterior wall myocardial infarction (MI). This is a sagittal view of the heart looking at the intraventricular septum. The left anterior descending (LAD) artery is coming down the front of the heart in an anterior wall MI, and the septal perforating branches supply the area of the septum in which the His bundle and right and left bundle branches run. Infranodal block in the setting of an anterior wall MI is potentially life-threatening because the escape rhythm is the ventricle itself, and complete asystole is statistically more likely to happen than when block in the AV node (AVN) occurs (although severe bradycardia or asystole can occur in both situations). (Modified from original artwork by Dr. Toshio Akiyama.)

the other hand, the prognosis for patients with anterior MI and complete AV block is poor, even in patients who are protected by a functioning temporary pacemaker. The cause of death is not bradycardia. Instead, death is a result of the extremely large infarction, overwhelming loss of myocardium, and cardiogenic shock. Injury to the infranodal conduction system is a marker for widespread necrosis. Despite the poor prognosis, some patients benefit from prophylactic pacing. Because it is difficult to predict which patients will benefit and which patients will not at the time the decision must be made, temporary pacemaker support is recommended for patients with anterior MI and the conduction problems outlined in the following paragraphs.

Bifascicular Block

New-onset bifascicular block (RBBB and either LAFB or left posterior fascicular block) is a harbinger of complete AV block in patients with acute MI and is an indication for prophylactic temporary pacing. If bifascicular block persists, permanent therapy is indicated. When it is transient, the indication for permanent pacing is less clear, although most clinicians recommend it in that setting.

It should be noted that changes in the QRS axis in patients with RBBB can be positively detected only with the 12-lead ECG. Axis shifts generally are either not apparent or are uninterpretable on inpatient telemetry systems, and therefore major axis shifts (fascicular blocks) can be overlooked. For this reason, any change in conduction seen on the monitor should prompt a 12-lead ECG to be obtained.

Left Bundle Branch Block

Most clinicians believe a temporary pacemaker should be placed in patients with new-onset left BBB. These patients, however, do not progress to complete heart block as frequently as those with RBBB and left anterior hemiblock. A common dilemma in patients with acute MI and BBB is determining whether the conduction abnormality is new or old. Previous ECGs often are not available. Clinically unstable patients may require a temporary pacemaker.

Right Bundle Branch Block

Right bundle branch block developing acutely with anterior MI does signify ischemia in the interventricular septum. Many physicians believe that prophylactic pacing is the safest choice for the individual patient, especially because the development of new LAFB or left posterior fascicular block may not be evident on routine telemetry. Ambulatory monitoring before discharge is advisable to exclude intermittent conduction disturbances or ventricular arrhythmias in these patients as well as those with other conduction abnormalities.

Anterior Fascicular Block

Isolated AFB does not commonly degenerate into complete AV block. Patients with AFB should be watched for the appearance of RBBB or complete left bundle branch block. Isolated posterior fascicular block (extreme right axis deviation) indicates a large area of injury in the interventricular septum because this is a broad structure anatomically. Isolated posterior fascicular block is rare and remains a controversial indication for a temporary pacemaker.

As noted previously, indications for pacemaker placement in patients after a MI are not absolute. Clinical judgment is required.

A similar anatomic event can occur with a relatively new procedure: ablation of the interventricular septum with alcohol installation. With this technique, patients with idiopathic hypertrophic subaortic stenosis are treated by instilling alcohol into some of the proximal septal perforators to destroy and cause scar formation in the interventricular septum, thus reducing the outflow gradient. These septal perforators also supply some of the infranodal conduction tissue, and one of the potential (but rare) complications of this technique is heart block.

Right Heart Catheter Placement in Patients with Left Bundle Branch Block

If placement of a Swan–Ganz catheter is anticipated in a patient with preexisting left BBB, one should be aware that, as catheters are maneuvered into the right-ventricular outflow tract, they pass by the portion of the interventricular septum, through which the right bundle passes. The patient is therefore at risk for temporary "bruising" of the right bundle, which is the only functioning bundle leading to transient (or, less commonly, permanent) complete AV block. Use of a temporary pacemaker in this setting should be considered.

Antitachycardia Therapy

Ventricular Tachycardia

Temporary pacing may be useful in the management of drug-resistant ventricular arrhythmias. Unfortunately, there is no panacea for resistant ventricular tachycardia, which usually occurs in a setting of severe left ventricular failure, often with associated myocardial ischemia. In selected patients who are resistant to drug therapy, however, overdrive suppression using a pacemaker either alone or in association with drugs may be helpful. This treatment has been especially effective for Torsade de pointes, a form of ventricular tachycardia with changing electric vectors, often occurring in a setting of prolonged QT interval and with toxicity resulting from quinidine, disopyramide, or other drugs that lengthen the QT interval. Overdrive suppression works by establishing a heart rate of 10 to 40 bpm above the resting heart rate. This shortens the QT interval and the refractory period of the ventricle. Ventricular ectopy often begins at an intrinsic heart rate that is fairly reproducible; that is, a patient may have ectopy begin at a heart rate of less than 60 bpm that no longer occurs when the heart rate increases to 90 bpm. By increasing the heart rate and shortening refractoriness, a rhythm is established that prevents ectopic ventricular beats. Generally, temporary atrial or ventricular pacing at 30 bpm above the resting rate is attempted. This approach is used much less commonly now that it has been learned that intravenous magnesium generally can terminate Torsade de pointes.

Another setting in which temporary ventricular pacing may benefit the patient is in the termination of sustained monomorphic ventricular tachycardia (SMMVT). In contrast to the mechanism of overdrive suppression and shortening of ventricular refractoriness described in regard to Torsade de pointes, SMMVT resulting from reentry often can be terminated by the introduction of properly timed premature ventricular beats or with short-duration burst ventricular pacing. In this situation, a fortuitously timed ventricular stimulus may produce a wave of excitation capable of causing bidirectional block within the pathway and terminate the circus movement of excitation. Although this measure is frequently effective in terminating SMMVT, one must be prepared for inadvertent tachycardia acceleration, which will result in LOC and the prompt need for cardioversion.

Some patients with ventricular arrhythmias benefit more from atrial pacing. Preservation of AV synchrony may enable toleration of more rapid pacing rates. In addition, the sequence of ventricular depolarization is physiologic when AV synchrony is maintained with atrial pacing. At times, this may be necessary to suppress ventricular ectopy. Altering the sequence of ventricular depolarization with ventricular pacing is advantageous in suppressing ventricular arrhythmias in some patients. Initially, the temporary pacemaker is placed in the ventricle with a rapid ventricular pacing to suppress ventricular tachycardia. If successful and tolerated by the patient, the temporary pacemaker lead is left in the ventricle. If the patient does not tolerate the lack of AV synchrony or if the ventricular pacing does not suppress the ventricular tachycardia, the ventricular lead is placed in the atrium and atrial pacing is attempted before efforts to achieve overdrive suppression are abandoned.

Atrial Tachycardia and Atrial Flutter

The principle of tachycardia termination for ectopic atrial tachycardia is similar to that for ventricular tachycardia. Overdrive suppression is especially useful for atrial flutter. This rhythm often occurs in acute illnesses, such as MI soon after cardiac surgery or exacerbation of pulmonary disease. Digitalis may be required to control the ventricular rate. Direct current cardioversion is usually successful in converting the rhythm. If the patient has received large doses of digitalis, however, ventricular arrhythmias may develop following countershock. Rapid atrial stimulation is a useful alternative. Care must be exercised to keep the catheter tip from moving to the right ventricle when the rapid pacing stimulus is applied; rapid ventricular pacing might stimulate ventricular tachycardia or fibrillation.

Drug-refractory paroxysmal supraventricular tachycardia may be approached in the same way. This condition is usually due to one of two tachyarrhythmias: AV nodal reentrant tachycardia or AV reentrant tachycardia involving an accessory pathway. By using either a properly timed premature atrial (or ventricular) stimulus or burst atrial pacing, the reentrant pathway may be penetrated by a premature wavefront of excitation and interrupt the reentry. This form of therapy is usually useful only in hospitalized patients who are planning to undergo elective radiofrequency catheter ablation of the slow AV nodal pathway or of the accessory pathway.

Most modern temporary transvenous pacemakers have a special setting that allows tachypacing up to several hundred beats per minute. Tachypacing is ineffective therapy for atrial fibrillation.

Other Uses for Temporary Pacemakers

Temporary pacemakers are used routinely in many other settings. After cardiac surgery, patients often have temporary pacemakers for both control of bradycardias and suppression of tachycardias.

Patients with asystole or profound and symptomatic bradycardia often need temporary pacemaker support while awaiting permanent pacemaker therapy. On occasion, treatment of supraventricular tachycardia with digoxin, beta-adrenergic blockers, or verapamil results in profound bradycardia that requires temporary pacing. As noted previously, such patients may need permanent pacemakers to tolerate the drug therapy necessary for control of supraventricular tachycardia.

The temporary pacemaker is useful in diagnosing cardiac arrhythmias. With a pacemaker in place and the distal lead attached to the V lead of the ECG, amplification of P waves and QRS complexes makes it possible to confirm the diagnosis of arrhythmias.

As noted earlier, temporary pacing is useful for testing the efficacy of pacing in the patient with marginal indications for permanent pacemaker therapy. The temporary pacemaker may help in predicting whether permanent pacing will be worthwhile. For example, in some patients with renal insufficiency, cerebral insufficiency, or congestive heart failure who also have bradycardia, temporary pacing may be helpful in determining whether a faster heart rate will result in improvement of these symptoms.

Often, the temporary pacemaker is used as a standby in high-risk clinical situations. For example, patients with conduction abnormalities may benefit from a temporary pacemaker during cardiac catheterization. Temporary pacing may be indicated for the patient who is severely symptomatic, particularly when a delay in permanent pacemaker insertion is anticipated. Temporary pacing also may be advisable for patients who must be transferred to another facility for insertion of the permanent pacemaker.

REFERENCES

Abi-Samra F, Maloney JD, Fouad-Tarazi FM, Castle LW. The usefulness of head-up tilt testing and hemodynamic investigations in the workup of syncope of unknown origin. *Pacing Clin Electrophysiol* 1988; 11:1202.

Anderson H, Nielsen J, Thomsen P, et al. Long-term follow-up of patients from a randomised trial of atrial versus ventricular pacing for sick-sinus syndrome. *Lancet* 1997;350:1210.

Anderson H, Thuesen L, Bagger, J, Vesterlund T, Thomsen P. Prospective randomised trial of atrial versus ventricular pacing in sick-sinus syndrome. *Lancet* 1994;344:1523.

Auricchio A., Klein H, Tockman B, et al. Transvenous biventricular pacing for heart failure: can the obstacles be overcome? *Am J Cardiol* 1999;83:136D.

Barold SS. ACC/AHA guidelines for implantation of cardiac pacemakers: how accurate are the definitions of atrioventricular conduction blocks? *Pacing Clin Electrophysiol* 1993;16:1221.

Behar S, Zissman E, Zion M, et al. Prognostic significance of second-degree atrioventricular block in inferior wall acute myocardial infarction. *Am J Cardiol* 1993;72:831.

Benditt D. Cardiac pacing for prevention of vasovagal syncope. *J Am Coll Cardiol* 1999;33:21.

Berger P, Ruocco N, Ryan T, et al. Incidence and prognostic implications of heart block complicating inferior myocardial infarction treated with thrombolytic therapy: results from TIMI II. *J Am Coll Cardiol* 1992;20:533.

Brignole M, Menozzi C, Gianfranchi L, et al. Assessment of Atrioventricular junction ablation and VVIR pacemaker versus pharmacological treatment in patients with heart failure and chronic atrial fibrillation. *Circulation* 1998;98:953.

Cairns J. Implantable cardioverter-defibrillators reduced mortality in patients resuscitated from ventricular arrhythmias. *ACP J Club* 1998;128:60.

Chokshi AB, Friedman HS, Malach M, et al. Impact of peer review in reduction of permanent pacemaker implantations. *JAMA* 1981;246:754.

Clark M, Sutton R, Ward D, et al. Recommendations for pacemaker prescription for symptomatic bradycardia. *Br Heart J* 1991;66:185.

Connolly SJ, Sheldon R, Roberts R, et al. Pacing therapy for vasovagal syncope: approach with caution. *J Am Coll Cardiol* 1999;33:16.

Connolly SJ, Sheldon R, Roberts R, et al. The North American Vasovagal Pacemaker Study (VPS), a randomized trial of permanent cardiac pacing for the prevention of vasovagal syncope. *J Am Coll Cardiol* 1999;33:16.

Cummins RO, Graves JR, Larsen MP, et al. Out-of-hospital transcutaneous pacing by emergency medical technicians in patients with asystolic cardiac arrest. *N Engl J Med* 1993;328:1377.

Delfaut P, Saksena S, Prakash A, Krol R. Long-term outcome of patients with drug-refractory atrial flutter and fibrillation after single- and dual-site right atrial pacing for arrhythmia prevention. *J Am Coll Cardiol* 1998;32:1900.

Dhingra RC, Palileo E, Strasberg B, et al. Significance of the HV interval in 517 patients with chronic bifascicular block. *Circulation* 1981;64:1265.

Fouad FM, Sitthisook S, Vanerio G, et al. Sensitivity and specificity of the tilt table test in young patients with unexplained syncope (Part I). *Pacing Clin Electrophysiol* 1993;16:394.

Freedman R. Controversial issues in the 1998 ACC/AHA Guidelines for Implantation of Cardiac Pacemakers. *ACC Current Journal Review* 1999;March/April:31.

Goldberg R, Zevallos J, Yarzebski J, et al. Prognosis of acute myocardial infarction complicated by complete heart block (the Worcester Heart Attack Study). *Am J Cardiol* 1992;69:1135.

Gregoratos G, Cheitlin M, Conill A, et al. ACC/AHA Guidelines for Implantation of Cardiac Pacemakers and Antiarrhythmia Devices. *J Am Coll Cardiol* 1998;31:1175.

Hayes D. Evolving indications for permanent pacing. *Am J Cardiol* 1999;83:161D.

Henderson M, Prabhu S. Syncope: current diagnosis and treatment. *Curr Probl Cardiol* 1997;22:243.

Hindman MC, Wagner GS, Jaro M, et al. The clinical significance of bundle branch block complicating acute myocardial infarction. 1. Clinical characteristics, hospital mortality, and one-year follow-up. *Circulation* 1978;58:679.

Hindman MC, Wagner GS, JaRo M, et al. The clinical significance of bundle branch block complicating acute myocardial infarction. 2. Indications for temporary and permanent pacemaker insertion. *Circulation* 1978;58:689.

Kapoor WN. Evaluation and management of the patient with syncope. *JAMA* 1992;268:2553.

Kass D, Chen C, Curry C, et al. Improved left ventricular mechanics from acute VDD pacing in patients with dilated cardiomyopathy and ventricular conduction delay. *Circulation* 1999;99:1567.

Lev M. The pathology of complete atrioventricular block. *Prog Cardiovasc Dis* 1964;6:317.

Linde C, Gadler F, Kappenberger L, Ryden L. Placebo effect of pacemaker implantation in obstructive hypertrophic cardiomyopathy. *Am J Cardiol* 1999;83:903.

Linzer M, Yang E, Estes M, et al. Diagnosing syncope, Part 1: value of history, physical examination, and electrocardiography. *Ann Intern Med* 1997;126:989.

Marshall H, Harris Z, Griffith M, Holder R, Gammage M. Prospective randomized study of ablation and pacing versus medical therapy for paroxysmal atrial fibrillation. *Circulation* 1999;99:1587.

McAnulty JH, Rahimtoola SH, Murphy E, et al. Natural history of "high-risk" bundle-branch block: final report of a prospective study. *N Engl J Med* 1982;307:137.

McComb J, Gribbin G. Effect of pacing mode on morbidity and mortality: update of clinical pacing trials. *Am J Cardiol* 1999;83:211D.

Menozzi C, Brignole M, Alboni P, et al. The natural course of untreated sick sinus syndrome and identification of the variables predictive of unfavorable outcome. *Am J Cardiol* 1998;82:1205.

Mills PS, Michnich ME. Managed care and cardiac pacing and electrophysiology. *Pacing Clin Electrophysiol* 1993;16:1746.

Prakash A, Saksena S, Hill M, et al. Acute effects of dual-site right atrial pacing in patients with spontaneous and inducible atrial flutter and fibrillation. *J Am Coll Cardiol* 1997;29:1007.

Rosenheck S, Bondy C, Weiss AT, Gotsman MS. Comparison between patients with and without reliable ventricular escape rhythm in the presence of long standing complete atrioventricular block. *Pacing Clin Electrophysiol* 1993;16:272.

Rosenqvist M. Atrial pacing for sick sinus syndrome. *Clin Cardiol* 1990;13:43.

Saksena S, Prakash A, Hill M, et al. Prevention of recurrent atrial fibrillation with chronic dual-site right atrial pacing. *J Am Coll Cardiol* 1996;28:687.

Schaumann A. Managing atrial tachyarrhythmias in patients with implantable cardioverter defibrillators. *Am J Cardiol* 1999;85:214D.

Sgarbossa EB, Pinski SL, Maloney JD. The role of pacing modality in determining long-term survival in the sick sinus syndrome. *Ann Intern Med* 1993;119:359.

Walter P. Greenspon A. Practical electrophysiology for the nonelectrophysiologist. *ACC Current Journal Review* 1997;Sept/Oct:76.

2

Pacemaker Technology

PERMANENT PACEMAKER TECHNOLOGY

The cardiac pacemaker is an electric circuit in which a battery provides electricity that travels through a conducting wire through the myocardium, stimulating the heart to beat ("capturing" the heart), and back to the battery, thus completing the circuit.

Definitions of Terms

Some simplified definitions and principles of electronics must be appreciated to discuss pacemaker technology.

Coulomb (C) is the unit of charge and is either positive or negative. One negative coulomb represents the charge of approximately 6.24×10^{18} electrons.

Ampere is the unit of electric current and represents a charge moving at the rate of 1 coulomb per second. It is often abbreviated *amp*. Because the current in a pacemaker is low, the units are usually in thousandths of an ampere, or milliamperes (mA). Current is abbreviated i or I.

Volt (V) is the unit of "electric pressure" or electromotive force that causes current to flow. Voltage can be thought of as the difference in potential energy between two points with an unequal electron population.

Resistance (R) is the opposition, present to varying degrees in all matter, to the flow of electric current.

Ohm (abbreviated Ω) is the unit of resistance. One ohm is the resistance that results in a current of 1 ampere when a potential of 1 volt is placed across the resistance.

Ohm's law states that voltage (V) is equal to current (i) times resistance (R): $V = iR$.

Impedance is a complex quantity having the dimensions of ohms. Whereas resistance applies only to idealized circuits with constant voltage and current and no capacitors, *impedance* is the proper term for the opposition to current flow in the pacing system. Complex mathematic methods exist for computing impedance, but we do not discuss these in this book. For our purposes, Ohm's law is adequate to describe the relationship among current, voltage, and impedance. In this text, the terms *impedance* and *resistance* will be used interchangeably, and the abbreviation *R* will be used for resistance or impedance.

Joule (J) is the fundamental unit of work or energy. In electric terms, in the pacing system, the energy released can be expressed as voltage × current × time = energy (in joules).

Watt (W) is the unit of power that is the rate at which work is done. One watt is 1 J per second, or voltage × current = watt.

Basic Principles of Pacing

An *electric circuit* must consist of a complete, closed loop for current to flow through it.

Conductors are materials with a relatively large number of free electrons and therefore pass an electric current well.

Insulators have few free electrons and therefore pass an electric current poorly.

A *capacitor* is a device made of two conductors separated by an insulator; it is used to store electrical charges.

A highly simplified circuit is shown in Figure 2-1. A battery is used to generate a force of 5 V. The circuit contains a 500-Ω resistor and the current, from Ohm's law, is 0.01 amp (or 10 mA). Figure 2-1 represents an oversimplification of the electric events during a pacing spike. In reality, the voltage, current, and impedance of a pacemaker system change throughout the delivery of the pacemaker spike.

Pacemaker Power Sources

General Characteristics of Pacemaker Batteries

The ideal pacemaker battery should be able to generate approximately 5 V, which exceeds the voltage normally required to stimulate the myocardium in patients, thus providing an adequate safety margin. The battery also should be

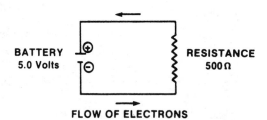

FLOW OF ELECTRONS

FIG. 2-1. Simple electric circuit. This closed loop circuit shows electrons flowing from the negative end of the circuit, through a wire, through a resistor, and back to the positive end of the battery. The driving force is 5 V, the resistance is 500 Ω, and the current is 10 mA. (Note that we are showing the actual direction of electron flow in this and subsequent figures. In standard electric circuit diagrams, current is traditionally and arbitrarily described as flowing from positive to negative.)

capable of being sealed hermetically. Many recalls of pacemakers by manufacturers have been caused by moisture intrusion into the unit; so hermetic sealing is important. Although *hermetic* means "airtight," we use the term in a stricter sense. *Hermeticity*, as defined by the pacing industry, is an extremely low rate of helium gas leakage from the sealed pacemaker container. The ideal pacemaker battery should have a low rate of *self-discharge*, meaning that it does not lose power when it is not being used, even over a period of several years. The battery should fail in a predictable manner so that an indicator such as rate change can be designed into the circuitry to warn the physician of impending battery failure and the need for replacement.

One of the most important characteristics of a pacemaker battery is its longevity in clinical use. A simple way to compare specific batteries is to note the number of electrons the battery can deliver over its lifetime. Because this number is large, the battery capacity is expressed in *ampere-hours*, which is the rate of delivery of electrons integrated over time. The ampere-hour rating depends on both the chemicals used in the battery and the physical size of the battery. Typical ampere-hour ratings for commercially used batteries are 1 to 3 ampere-hours. Theoretically, a battery with a rating of 3 ampere-hours is superior to a battery with a rating of 1 or 2 ampere-hours, but this type of comparison is oversimplified. The voltage at which the battery operates is also important, the size of the battery is important clinically, and the theoretically deliverable energy may be more than the actual deliverable energy when a battery is in a patient and in use over a period of years. Thus, although the ratings are potentially useful, the possibility of an inappropriate comparison exists.

The main purpose of the pacemaker's battery power is to stimulate the heart with the pacemaker spike. In demand units, the pacemaker must sense the patient's relatively weak QRS signal requiring amplification. Sensing is not a passive process and does require a small amount of power. A small amount of power also is required for the timing device in the pacemaker.

Testing batteries by battery specialists is extremely important in predicting battery performance and is a major thrust in the industry. Recent trends in battery technology have involved decreasing the size of the battery. Much of the reduction in the size of the pacemaker battery has been due to more efficient electronics in the pacemaker generator and more efficient lead systems, both of which allow pacing with safe threshold at lower energies and therefore allow longer battery life or smaller batteries.

How a Pacemaker Battery Works

Because the most commonly used power source in the United States is now the lithium iodine battery, we will use it as an example of how a battery works. All batteries consist of three basic components: a material that gives off electrons (the *anode*), a material that takes up electrons (the *cathode*), and an ionic conductor that separates the anode and cathode (the *electrolyte*). The electrode reactions of the battery may be represented as follows:

$$2Li \rightarrow 2Li^+ + 2e^- \text{ (anode reaction)}$$

$$2Li^+ + 2e^- + I_2 \rightarrow 2LiI \text{ (cathode reaction)}$$

$$2Li + I_2 \rightarrow 2LiI \text{ (overall reaction)}$$

where Li = lithium, e = electron, I = current, and LiI = lithium iodide.

In this example, the lithium at the anode *ionizes* (loses an electron) and migrates as a positively charged ion through the electrolyte toward the cathode. The electrolyte is the lithium iodide that is formed continuously by the reaction between lithium and iodine. Electrons are left behind at the anode, which therefore becomes negatively charged relative to the other electrode (cathode). If the two electrodes then are connected by a conductive pathway (for example, a pacing wire in a patient), electrons can flow from one end of the battery to the other. The definitions of anode and cathode for a battery and for current flow in a circuit are opposites. The anode of a battery is the negative end of the battery, whereas in an electric circuit, the same negative electrode is called the *cathode*. Because this is rather confusing, after this brief discussion of batteries, we will use these terms only as they apply to the total circuit and not to the battery.

The LiI formed during the use of the battery is a solid that gradually increases the separation between the lithium and the iodine in the battery. This separation slowly causes the voltage of the battery to drop, even though both lithium and iodine remain in the battery. The battery does not run down because of depletion of chemicals; instead, the internal resistance of the battery rises, causing the voltage to drop. This concept is of clinical relevance because companies make pacemakers that are capable of giving noninvasive readings of the internal resistance of the lithium iodine battery as an index of battery depletion.

Types of Pacemaker Batteries

The *lithium anode battery* has become the most commonly used pacing power source. Several types are either in use or under investigation. The lithium iodine battery generates 2.8 V at body temperature. Use of a voltage doubler in the circuit can raise the pacing voltage to approximately 5.0. (The doubler is not 100% efficient.) Estimating the life of the lithium iodine battery is difficult because modifications have been made in their manufacture, and current drain varies considerably in individual patients. A realistic estimate of the life of contemporary lithium iodine batteries is 4 to 10 years. It should be emphasized that battery life does not equal pacemaker life, because problems with circuitry or the lead system may cause pacemaker failure despite a functioning battery. One major influence on battery life is its physical size, a consideration that is sometimes clinically important. A small, thin lithium iodine generator with an estimated life of approximately 4 years (assuming complete pacing) may be reasonable in an elderly, thin patient who has a short life expectancy or in whom the pacemaker is expected to be used only intermittently. A larger, heavier unit with an estimated life of 8 years or longer is more reasonable in a patient who has a longer life expectancy and in whom generator size is not a major concern.

The more frequent use of DDD pacemakers, which in many patients leads to two pacemaker spikes per heartbeat instead of one, drains a battery more rapidly. Also, some of the sensor technology used for rate-responsive pacing leads to earlier battery depletion. These factors complicate the estimate of battery life.

The *lithium iodine battery* has become so widely used that there is a tendency to equate the lithium iodine battery with all pacemaker batteries. Other lithium batteries have been used as well (specifically, the lithium cupric sulfide battery and the lithium silver chromate battery). These batteries have different characteristics and have been useful in the past but are used less commonly, if ever, today.

A different type of lithium battery that is valuable, however, is the *lithium vanadium silver pentoxide battery*, which is used in the implantable defibrillator. This type of battery, rather than a lithium iodine battery, is used for the implantable defibrillator because of the need for rapid discharge from the battery to supply relatively high-power requirements for repeated shocks to the heart. The lithium iodine discharge would be inappropriately slow. With different batteries, different end-of-life characteristics occur, but in general the lithium batteries have been quite effective and have dominated the pacemaker market.

The *zinc mercuric oxide battery* was the power source most commonly used in the early years after pacemakers were introduced and is of historical interest. The battery has a voltage of only 1.35 V; therefore, five or six batteries usually were placed in series to provide adequate voltage for pacing. Compared with the currently used lithium batteries, the zinc mercuric oxide battery has a relatively short life of 1 to 5 years, it cannot be hermetically sealed because it produces gas with use, and it is capable of sudden failure. Because of these problems, it is no longer implanted.

Nuclear-powered pacemakers were first used clinically around 1970. Since then, a few thousand have been implanted. Despite a long life expectancy, the nuclear battery has some disadvantages compared with the lithium battery and is seldom used. Nuclear batteries cost more than lithium batteries, controversy exists over what constitutes safe and acceptable radiation exposure to the patient, and regulations about follow-up of the patient are necessarily strict to minimize the chance of environmental contamination with radioactive material.

Cadmium nickel oxide batteries are externally rechargeable batteries that require recharging every few weeks. They have been used for several years but have not gained widespread acceptance.

Pacemaker Circuitry

The microprocessor-based technology that revolutionized the computer industry also has revolutionized the pacemaker industry. The semiconductors used in pacemakers allow handling of complex information in a small space at a relatively low cost with little expenditure of energy, little generation of heat, and a high degree of reliability. One of the reasons that semiconductor circuitry is both more complex and more reliable than the older "discrete component" technology is that few welded metal-to-metal connections are required. In a circuit, the fewer welded connections present, the more reliable it is. If a modern multiprogrammable pacemaker were constructed using transistor technology, it would be at least as large as a television set.

Some of the terms used in describing pacemaker circuitry are not widely familiar and are briefly explained below.

A *semiconductor* is a crystal (usually silicon, which is normally a nonconductor) that has had its crystal structure deliberately contaminated with other atoms. (This process is referred to as *doping.*) These atoms replace silicon atoms in the structure of the crystal but have one valence electron more or less than the four in silicon that are necessary for proper binding. As a result, the doped crystal tends to accept or donate electrons easily from an added atom.

The abbreviation *CMOS* is used often in pacemaker advertisements to describe the unit's circuitry and stands for "complementary metallic oxide semiconductor." When an area in a semiconductor that tends to accept electrons is next to an area that tends to donate electrons, they are *complementary*; electrons can flow in an unidirectional current at low voltage with little generation of heat. The complex CMOS technology is extremely compact and operates at low energy. In the future, other types of semiconductor technology may be used in pacemakers.

Large-scale integration (LSI) is a nonspecific term that refers to the technology that produces high-density circuits with the capacity of having thousands of components in an area of a few square millimeters.

The semiconductor chip or chips are only one portion of the pacemaker circuitry, which also contains resistors, capacitors, and other components. The process of combining these components into a single complex circuit is referred to as *hybridization.* Figure 2-2 depicts a hybrid circuit.

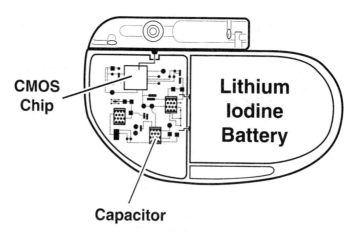

FIG. 2-2. Hybrid circuit of a programmable pacemaker. This circuit is connected to a lithium battery and the entire system is hermetically sealed in a metal covering. It then can be connected to a fitting for the pacing wire connector, thus forming the complete pacemaker generator. (*CMOS,* complementary metallic oxide semiconductor.)

Other terms used in describing pacemaker circuits include *digital technology* and *analog technology*. In digital technology, information is processed by turning switches on or off. It is reliable and energy efficient and may be used in the timing circuit and programming circuits. In analog technology, information is processed by regulating the amount of current or voltage in a system; for example, the sensing circuit may use analog technology to sense the amplitude of the patient's QRS complex.

The general principles of the programmable circuitry of an idealized pacemaker are discussed in Chapter 4.

The Pacemaker Lead

The pacing lead conducts electricity from the pacemaker generator to the heart (and, in the bipolar system, back to the other pole of the pacemaker generator to complete the circuit). Because the heart beats approximately 40 million times per year, the lead must be resistant to fracture to withstand this chronic flexure. Usually the wire (or wires, in the bipolar system) is made of a metal alloy to allow good conductivity, is fatigue resistant, is coiled to increase flexibility, and is multifilar to provide redundancy within the lead.

The wire must be insulated from the body, and if the lead is bipolar, both wires must be insulated from each other, usually with Silastic or polyurethane; only the metal tip or electrode is exposed. Some clinical differences exist between Silastic and polyurethane coating. Polyurethane tends to allow a smaller size, and be more slippery, and some polyurethane leads have demonstrated stress cracking in the surface, sometimes of clinical significance. The Silastic leads tend to be somewhat larger and less slippery and have proven durability. Newer types of insulation are overcoming these differences.

Numerous styles of permanent leads are available. A schematic description of an old transvenous lead is shown in Figure 2-3. This lead has separate connectors for the wires that go to the tip electrode and the ring electrode. The wires are side by side and insulated from each other and from the body. The exposed metal tips appear stippled. Figure 2-4 demonstrates a bipolar lead with a coiled three-strand wire (for redundancy if one strand should fracture) going to the exposed tip and a separate wire going to the metal band or ring electrode approximately 1 to 2 cm behind the tip. The end of the lead is flanged with plastic "wings" to facilitate entrapment of the lead in the trabeculae of the right ventricle.

Figure 2-5 demonstrates a more modern-type lead. The connections to the positive and negative ends of the battery are now "in line." (Compare with Fig. 2-3, in which the electrodes and wires are separate from each other.) These are placed in line to facilitate placement into the pacemaker head. This design is called the *International Standard I* (IS-I). The wires are coaxial, meaning that one wire is coiled inside the other and they are insulated from each other. If the wire is made unipolar with only one wire going to the tip, the metal connectors appear identical and there is a "dummy" metal connector for the band area so

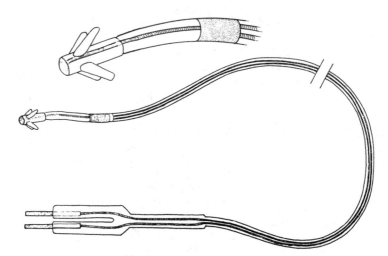

FIG. 2-3. A hypothetical bipolar lead of the type that is no longer used. It does, however, present a simpler explanation of the bipolar lead. In this case, there are two connecting electrodes for both the tip and the band electrode. The wires run side by side and are insulated from each other and from the body. One wire goes to the "band" electrode proximally, and the other goes to the tip electrode at the distal portion. The stippled areas in this figure indicate exposed metal. This is purely for diagrammatic purposes. Current leads are "coaxial," with one wire wound inside the other; however, the wires still are insulated from each other and from the body. The wires are no longer used side by side because they are more bulky and potentially more easily subjected to stress fractures. The two connecting electrodes in a bipolar lead, as noted in Fig. 2-4, are placed "in line" rather than side by side.

that either a unipolar or bipolar connector will fit into the same pacing head. This could be a source of confusion to someone inexperienced in pacemaker placement.

The atrial J lead has become popular for transvenous atrial pacing. The lead is straightened with a stylet and advanced to the right atrium. The stylet is withdrawn, and the lead is lodged in the right atrial appendage (Fig. 2-6).

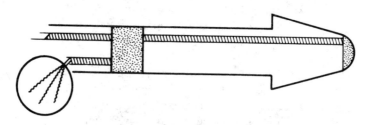

FIG. 2-4. Detail of a bipolar lead. The wires are triple-wound (tri-filar) helical coils. One goes to the exposed metal tip and the other to the exposed metal ring approximately 3 cm back from the tip. The wires are insulated from the body and from each other by a Silastic or polyurethane coating.

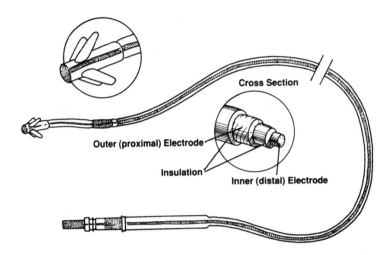

FIG. 2-5. Permanent pacemaker lead of a more modern type. The end of this bipolar lead, which is inserted into the pacemaker, has two electrodes "in line." The two wires are "coaxial," meaning that one wire is coiled inside the other with insulation between them, and the wires are insulated from the body (see inset).

An epicardial lead is shown in Figure 2-7. This particular model is a screw-in electrode that uses the tip of the screw as the pacing tip. It is the most common type of epicardial wire used for transthoracic pacing. Care must be taken to ensure that the pacing tip does not penetrate the myocardium entirely, resulting in loss of contact with excitable myocardium.

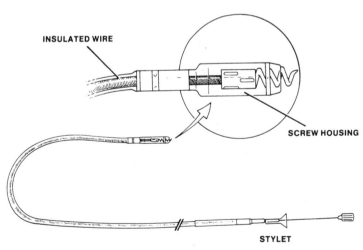

FIG. 2-6. Permanent pacing lead, screw-in type. The screw-in lead can be used in either the ventricle or the atrium. It is an active fixation lead. The stylet can be curved to guide the pacemaking lead into the proper position and then can be removed. The screws can be turned so that they exit from the screw housing area and turn into the myocardium for permanent fixation.

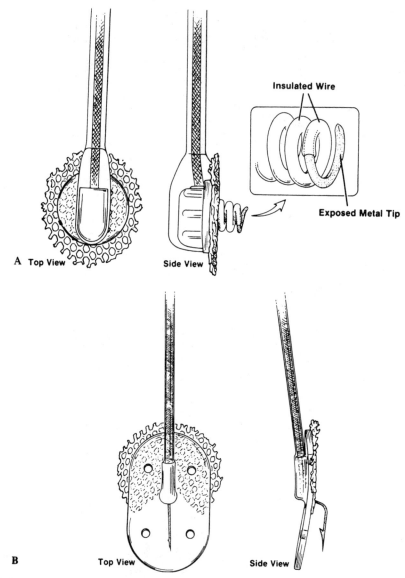

A Top View   Side View

Insulated Wire

Exposed Metal Tip

B   Top View   Side View

FIG. 2-7. A: Epicardial screw-in electrode. During surgery, the heart is exposed, and the electrode is screwed into the myocardium. Only the tip of the screw is exposed because the area of the exposed electrode should not be too large if effective pacing is to occur. Care must be taken that the tip does not penetrate the wall and lose contact with the myocardium. **B:** Another type of myocardial lead often used for atrial pacing.

Unipolar Versus Bipolar Pacing

Pacing systems are either unipolar or bipolar. A transvenous bipolar pacemaker is diagrammed in Figure 2-8. The battery is implanted in the chest wall, and a lead containing two wires connects the battery to the apex of the right ventricle. The pacemaker battery generates current that passes through the wire attached to the negative end of the battery to the myocardium and back through the other wire to the positive terminal, thus completing the circuit.

The distal electrode usually is attached to the negative terminal (cathode) because the heart is generally more easily stimulated if electrons travel from the distal electrode, which usually has the best myocardial contact, to the proximal electrode. In electrophysiologic studies, this cathodal stimulation depolarizes a cell slightly more easily than anodal stimulation. Reversing polarity of the leads and connecting the positive pole (anode) to the tip electrode, however, sometimes results in a lower stimulation threshold.

A unipolar pacemaker is shown in Figure 2-9. The term *unipolar* is misleading because all electric circuits have two poles. In the unipolar system, however, the lead connecting the battery to the right ventricular apex contains only one wire. Electrons travel through the insulated wire to the exposed tip (the cathode)

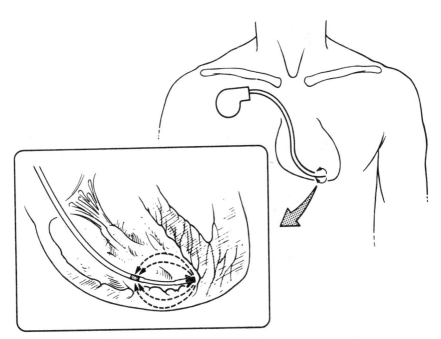

FIG. 2-8. Bipolar pacemaker. During the brief pacemaker spike, electrons flow from the negative end of the generator through an insulated wire toward the negative electrode (cathode) and to the endocardium. Electricity then travels approximately 2 cm through tissue to the other pacemaker wire (the anode or band electrode) and back to the positive end of the battery.

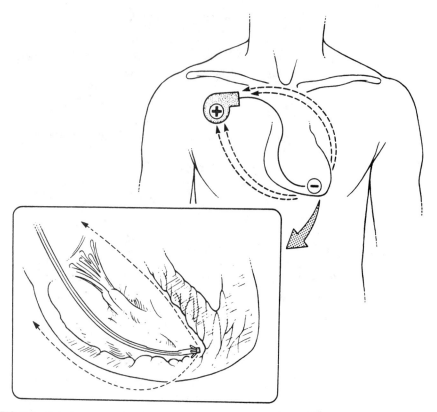

FIG. 2-9. Unipolar pacemaker. During the brief pacemaker spike, electrons flow from the negative end of the pacemaker battery through insulated wire to the exposed wire tip (cathode) and to the endocardium. Electricity then flows through the heart muscle, stimulating it, and through the chest tissue back to the wall of the pacemaker (the anode) that is connected to the positive end of the circuit.

and back through myocardial and chest tissue to the metal wall of the pacemaker generator (the anode), which is internally attached to the positive pole of the battery in the generator. If only one wall of the unipolar pacemaker generator conducts electricity, that side is placed in the chest wall facing outward, away from the pectoralis muscle, to minimize the chance of the electric current causing pectoral muscle stimulation.

Electrocardiograms obtained from a patient with a bipolar pacemaker and a patient with a unipolar pacemaker are shown in Figs. 2-10 and 2-11, respectively. Both pacemakers are functioning normally. Note that the pacemaker spike caused by the bipolar unit is smaller than the one caused by the unipolar pacemaker because the electricity travels a shorter distance through body tissue in the bipolar model. Each of these endocardial leads is in the right ventricular apex. Note also the approximate, deeply negative QRS complexes in leads II, III, and

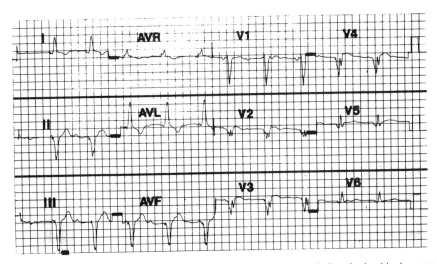

FIG. 2-10. Bipolar electrocardiogram done on a patient with a normally functioning bipolar pacemaker with the transvenous endocardial electrode appropriately placed in the apex of the right ventricle. Note the small pacemaker spike compared with the unipolar pacemaker in Figure 2-11 and the appropriate left bundle branch block and left axis deviation pattern.

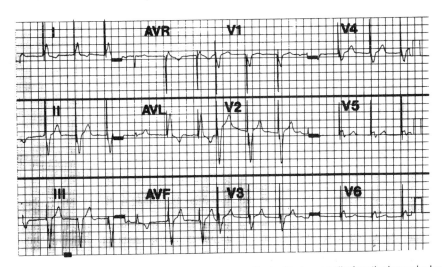

FIG. 2-11. Unipolar electrocardiograph done on a patient with a normally functioning unipolar pacemaker with the transvenous endocardial electrode appropriately placed in the apex of the right ventricle. Note the large pacemaker spike compared with the bipolar pacemaker in Figure 2-10 and the appropriate left bundle branch block and left axis deviation pattern.

AVF as the heart is depolarized from apex to base and in the anterior precordial leads as the heart is depolarized from front to back.

In general, the bipolar lead appears to have some advantage over the unipolar lead. Some of the differences between unipolar and bipolar pacing systems are itemized herein.

Size

The unipolar electrode is, with only one wire, slightly smaller. It may be useful if the vein used is small. Coaxial bipolar leads with one wire coiled inside the other have minimized the size differences. On the other hand, a unipolar pacing electrode needs insulation around one wire only; because it needs only half the insulation, there may be a slight reliability advantage (less chance of an insulation break).

Voltage Threshold

The current threshold is identical for both unipolar and bipolar pacemakers, but the voltage threshold tends to be 30% higher in the bipolar system because impedance tends to be higher in the bipolar system. (Recall that according to Ohm's law, $i = V/R$, and if resistance increases, the voltage also must increase to maintain the same current.) Although the electric current in the bipolar system has a shorter distance to travel in the body, the bipolar anode (usually the ring electrode) is much smaller than in the unipolar system (in which the anode is one metal wall of the pacemaker generator or the entire generator). A larger anode size results in slightly lower resistances and more than offsets any effect of the greater distance between the cathode and anode. The effect of the size of the anode on resistance is related to polarization resistance (see Chapter 3). This difference in voltages is minimized with the larger band electrode and is not a clinically important difference.

Extra Wire

The bipolar electrode contains two wires. If one wire fractures, the pacemaker sometimes can be converted to a unipolar system, thus avoiding electrode replacement. If a coaxial system is used, in the bipolar system, one wire is coiled inside the other and the lead may be somewhat stiffer than in a unipolar system. One potential problem with the bipolar system is that the two wires need to be insulated from each other. If an insulation break were to occur between the two wires, it would cause a "short," and electricity would travel around in a circuit up to the generator and down to the area of insulation break and not pace the heart.

Sensing

The unipolar pacemaker is somewhat more sensitive to interference from external signals, such as muscle contraction or electromagnetic interference, whereas the bipolar pacemaker may be more likely to fail to sense QRS complexes properly. Improvements in sensing characteristics have minimized this difference between the two types of pacemakers.

Skeletal Muscle Stimulation

In the unipolar unit, current travels through the heart and chest wall and occasionally may stimulate the pectoral muscle.

Stimulus Artifact Amplitude

The pacemaker spike is larger in the unipolar system and can distort the ECG baseline. This distortion can give the impression, to anyone unfamiliar with the unipolar system, that the spike is followed by a QRS complex, when in fact it is not. In contrast, the bipolar spike can be more difficult to see on a rhythm strip. A smaller spike size in the bipolar system may be of particular benefit in an automatic implantable cardioverter-defibrillator (ICD) device, which senses the patient's intrinsic QRS complex. The unipolar spike, for instance, might be sensed as a QRS complex, even if the patient is in ventricular fibrillation and the device may not fire. This is one technical consideration that needs to be considered in designing combination defibrillators and pacemaker systems.

Damage

The bipolar system may be less susceptible to damage in a patient requiring defibrillation.

Surface Area of the Electrode Tip

The ideal surface area of the electrode tip has been investigated. With smaller electrode tips, the electricity delivered to the heart is more concentrated and the heart more readily stimulated to contract; from that viewpoint, therefore, smaller tips are better (Fig. 2-12). As the tip becomes smaller, however, resistance to the transmission of electricity increases (mainly the polarization resistance discussed in the next chapter), and if a tip is too small, the increased polarization resistance results in poor sensing of the patient's QRS complexes. Electrodes used in the past often had tip areas of approximately 50 mm^2; present-day electrode tips usually measure 8 to 12 mm^2 in area, a size that represents a compromise between two opposing effects.

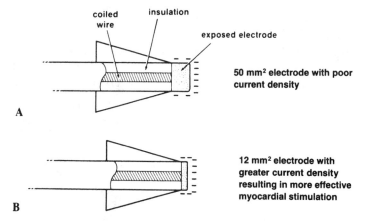

FIG. 2-12. Current density. **A:** An older-model electrode tip of 50-mm^2 surface area has poor current density. **B:** When the same charge is sent through a 12-mm^2 electrode, the same number of electrons is more concentrated and stimulates the myocardium more effectively. For myocardial stimulation, the smaller electrode is the better; however, when electrode area is much less than 8-12 mm^2, the sensing ability of the electrode is impaired. (Polarization resistance rises, as discussed in Chapter 3.)

TEMPORARY PACEMAKER TECHNOLOGY

Battery and Generator

The technology of temporary pacing is much simpler than that of permanent pacing because size, longevity, and hermeticity are not important. Most temporary generators use a standard 9-V alkaline battery that can be bought at any drugstore. This voltage is increased by special circuitry so that the voltage output is approximately 15 V, as opposed to most permanent pacemakers, which have a maximum of 5 V.

One difference between temporary pacemaker generators and most permanent pacemaker generators is that the temporary pacemaker provides a constant current rather than a constant voltage. This important concept is discussed in more detail in Chapter 3.

Lead

Temporary pacemaker leads often are insulated wires that are stiffer than permanent pacemaker electrodes. Balloon-tipped leads are available for emergency use, as are transthoracic leads. We prefer disposable leads because, with resterilization and reuse, small cracks that are not visible through the insulation may cause intermittent fractures in the wire. A cable usually is used to connect the generator to the lead.

Every nurse and physician who works in an emergency room or coronary care unit, or who is responsible for attending cardiac arrests, should understand electric safety considerations, know how to connect the circuitry for bipolar and unipolar pacing, and know how to change bipolar to unipolar pacing.

Because the bipolar circuit is the more easily understood and more foolproof, we attempt to keep only bipolar units on our emergency carts. The circuitry is exactly analogous to the permanent pacemaker circuitry in Fig. 2-8. Electricity leaves the battery and travels down the wire connected to the negative terminal, through the myocardium, and back through the wire connected to the positive terminal, thus completing the circuit. Little confusion about positive and negative exists with bipolar pacemakers because the lead connections usually are labeled. Even a person who knows nothing about electric circuits can realize they must be connected to the positive and the negative battery terminals. The distal electrode is labeled *negative* because, as mentioned earlier, the empiric observation has been made that lower pacing thresholds often are obtained if electrons flow from distal to proximal electrode rather than vice versa. If obtaining a good threshold is a problem, however, the leads can be reversed by attaching the proximal wire to the negative terminal and allowing electrons to flow from proximal to distal tips. An occasional patient will pace better with that type of connection, and even if the leads are reversed in the excitement of an emergency, usually no clinical problem results.

The temporary unipolar system may confuse someone unfamiliar with pacemakers but is analogous to the permanent unipolar system shown in Figure 2-9. A single electrode is passed to the heart and (usually) connected to the negative electrode. Electrons pass through the wire and the heart; then, to complete the circuit, they must pass to the skin, where a metal clamp, needle, or wire suture has been attached to a wire connected to the positive terminal of the generator. An example is shown in Fig. 2-13. Again, because the bipolar system is less confusing and does not involve the exposed skin connection, we use bipolar wires for temporary pacing.

A bipolar pacemaker can be converted easily to a unipolar pacemaker by connecting either the distal or proximal electrode to (usually) the negative pole of the pacemaker, leaving the other electrode unused. (The tip should be covered with a rubber glove so it cannot accidentally short-circuit the pacing circuit.) The positive pole is connected to a wire suture, needle, or metal plate in firm contact with the skin of the patient.

Safety Procedures

Temporary pacemakers present several safety problems that are not associated with permanent pacemakers. A major one is the fact that a wire exposed to the environment is directly in contact with the endocardium. For this reason, among others, all electrical equipment in an intensive or coronary care unit must be grounded and inspected regularly to eliminate the possibility of a microshock causing ventricular fibrillation. The battery, generator, and terminals must be protected against moisture. Terminals must be protected against conducting

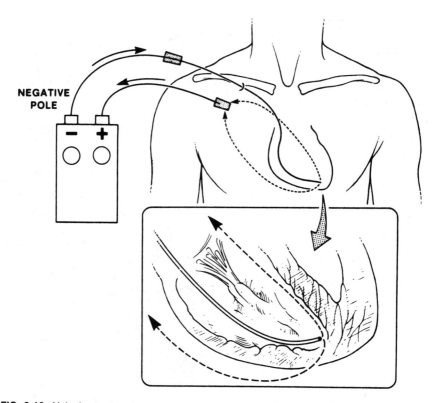

NEGATIVE POLE

FIG. 2-13. Unipolar temporary pacing circuit. The pacing wire has been advanced through a right subclavian vein to the right ventricular apex. Electrons flow from the negative pole through the myocardium to stimulate it, through body tissue to an alligator clamp attached to the skin, then through the wire connected to the positive terminal, thus completing the circuit. Good electric contact must exist between the clamp and the skin. The alligator clamp is used only briefly while positioning the electrode and determining threshold. Later, a more stable contact such as a wire suture must be used.

material that could short-circuit the system. Systematic testing of batteries and reusable pacing wires and cables must be performed. Usually, this task is the responsibility of the hospital's engineering department, which has access to ampmeters and other testing equipment.

REFERENCES

Baker RG Jr, Falkenberg EN. Bipolar versus unipolar issues in DDD pacing (Part II). *Pacing Clin Electrophysiol* 1984;7:1178.

Breivik K, Ohm O-J, Engedal H. Long-term comparison of unipolar and bipolar pacing and sensing, using a new multiprogrammable pacemaker system (Part I). *Pacing Clin Electrophysiol* 1983;6:592.

de Voogt W. Pacemaker leads: performance and progress. *Am J Cardiol* 1999;83:187D.

Furman S, Garvey J, Hurzeler P. Pulse duration variation and electrode size as factors in pacemaker longevity. *J Thorac Cardiovasc Surg* 1975;69:382.

Furman S, Parker B, Escher DJW, Solomon N. Endocardial threshold of cardiac response as a function of electrode surface area. *J Surg Res* 1968;8:161.

Hill WE, Murray A, Bourke JP, et al. Minimum energy for cardiac pacing. *Clin Phys Physiol Meas* 1988;9:41.

Jeffrey K, Parsonnet V. Cardiac pacing, 1960–1985, a quarter century of medical and industrial innovation. *Circulation* 1998;97:1978.

Mugica J. Progress and development of cardiac pacing electrodes (Part I). *Pacing Clin Electrophysiol* 1990;13:1558.

Parsonnet V, Berstein AD, Perry GY. The nuclear pacemaker: is renewed interest warranted? *Am J Cardiol* 1990;66:837.

Phillips R, Frey M, Martin RO. Long-term performance of polyurethane pacing leads: mechanisms of design-related failures (Part II). *Pacing Clin Electrophysiol* 1986;9:1166.

Schuchert A, Kuck K-H. Influence of internal current and pacing current on pacemaker longevity. *Pacing Clin Electrophysiol* 1994;17:13.

Zoll PM. Noninvasive temporary cardiac pacing. *J Electrophysiol* 1987;1:156.

Zoll PM, Zoll RH, Falk RH, et al. External noninvasive temporary cardiac pacing: clinical trials. *Circulation* 1985;71:937.

3

Electrophysiology of Pacing

PERMANENT PACEMAKER ELECTROPHYSIOLOGY

Polarization Resistance

Resistance is opposition to the flow of electric current, and one aspect of cardiac pacing that often confuses the beginner is that resistance or impedance is not static during a pacemaker spike; the resistance increases with time. The rise of polarization resistance with time occurs because electricity is being conducted through a wire, through an electrolyte solution (i.e., the body), and then back through another wire. The tip of a bipolar wire is negatively charged, and the ring or band electrode is positively charged. Positive ions in the electrolyte solution begin to travel toward the negatively charged metal surface, and negative ions in the solution travel toward the positive electrode. This polarization effect resists the flow of electricity through the circuit. The longer the current is turned on, the greater is the extent of polarization (as shown in Fig. 3-1); hence, the polarization resistance increases with time. When the electricity is turned off, these polarized ions stay apart for a brief period, and this creates a transient current called *after-potential*. In effect, the polarization has created a brief "battery" with separation of the positive and negative ions.

The polarization effect becomes less prominent as the area of exposed metal surface increases. This inverse relationship explains why the impedance in a unipolar pacemaker is lower than in a bipolar pacemaker. Although in the unipolar system electricity must travel a longer distance through the body, the electrolyte solution that comprises intracellular and extracellular fluid is a good conductor of electricity and is not a major source of resistance. The distal electrode tips are small in both the unipolar and bipolar systems; however, the large exposed metal plate of the unipolar anode (as opposed to the small surface area of the bipolar anode) causes the polarization resistance to be lower in the unipolar system.

As mentioned in Chapter 2, the smaller the electrode tip, the more concentrated the electric charge. With more concentrated charge, the heart muscle can be stimulated with lower energy levels. If this were the only consideration, the

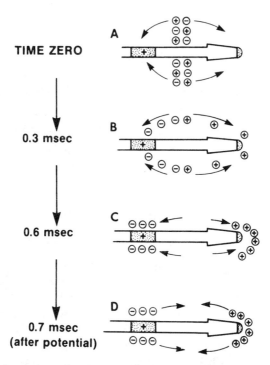

FIG. 3-1. Polarization resistance and after-potential. **A,B:** At the beginning of the pacemaker spike, ions have not migrated to the oppositely charged metal surface in any significant number. **C:** By the end of the 0.6-msec spike, the polarization of the ions has progressed, and the buildup of oppositely charged ions at the metal electrodes opposes the flow of electricity through the circuit and increases resistance (impedance) with time. **D:** Once the pacemaker spike ends, these polarized ions cause a small sensed current (after-potential) before they mix and become electrically neutral.

smallest tip would be the best; in fact, electrode tips are now much smaller than they were initially. If an electrode tip is made too small, however, the increase in polarization resistance becomes a problem, especially with sensing. In sensing, the electricity generated by the heart itself must travel through the pacemaker circuit to be sensed; because the signal generated is a fairly weak one, its further attenuation by polarization resistance may result in nonsensing. Present-day pacemaker electrodes have exposed metal pacing tips that are as small as practical to permit maximum charge concentration without causing sensing problems.

Constant-voltage and Constant-current Pacing

Most permanent pacemakers are *constant-voltage pacemakers* because the voltage remains fairly constant throughout the pacemaker spike. In practice, no permanent pacemaker can maintain an exactly even voltage throughout the pacing spike. Voltage at the leading edge of the spike is higher than at the trailing edge because the capacitor in the pacemaker is necessarily small and cannot store a charge large enough to maintain a strictly constant voltage (this drop in voltage is referred to as *tilt* and is of greater clinical importance in implantable cardioverter defibrillators). Because of this limitation, the more accurate term *constant-voltage capacitor-coupled pacemaker* is sometimes used. Figure 3-2 compares a constant-voltage spike with a constant-voltage capacitor-coupled spike, and Figure 3-3 describes a single constant-voltage capacitor-coupled pacemaker spike in terms of typical charges in voltage, impedance, and current.

Another type of pacemaker is the *constant-current pacemaker*, which is designed to provide a constant current despite variation in impedance. As impedance rises, voltage is increased to maintain a constant current. (Again recall that according to Ohm's law, i = V/R.) The increase in voltage to maintain a constant current in the face of rising impedance is limited by the voltage capacity of the pacemaker. For example, a pacemaker programmed to deliver a current of 10 mA with a 5-V battery could maintain a constant current of 5 mA only if the impedance of the system remained below 500 Ω. Once impedance rises above 500 Ω, the battery simply generates its maximum power of 5 V and acts like a constant-voltage pacemaker. Because of this limitation, the more accurate term *constant-current voltage-limited pacemaker* is used often (Fig. 3-4).

Constant-current pacing in the past was used in some permanent pacemakers, and it is used in almost all external pacemakers for temporary pacing. The power

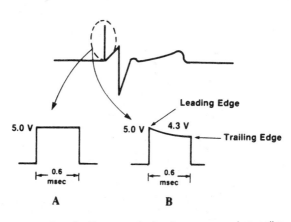

FIG. 3-2. Pacemaker spike. **A:** True constant-voltage pacemaker spike (not present in implantable permanent pacemaker). **B:** Constant-voltage capacitor-coupled spike. The spike is seen on the surface electrocardiogram (*ECG*) as a thin line, but when magnified on an oscilloscope, it has a precise time duration or width (in this case, 0.6 msec) and voltage. The changes in pulse duration that are programmable cannot be detected on a routine ECG and require a special device to be measured. The voltage drop in the spike labeled B occurs because the energy is being delivered from a capacitor discharge and a constant voltage cannot be maintained by the capacitor.

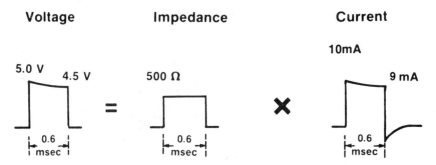

FIG. 3-3. Constant-voltage capacitor-coupled pacemaker spike. The changes in voltage, imped-ance, and current are shown for a single pacemaker spike. Note the slight drop in voltage from leading edge to trailing edge in the pacemaker spike. The impedance stays relatively constant in this example. Because of the drop in voltage, the current also drops from 10 mA at the begin-ning of the spike to 9 mA at the end of the spike. (A small, transient, negative current is seen on the current spike because of after-potential; see Fig. 3-1.)

source of most external pacemakers supplies approximately 15 V; so a true con-stant current can be maintained in the face of considerable increases in imped-ance. Batteries in these temporary pacemakers are fairly large and have a short life span compared with those in permanent pacemakers, but neither size nor life span is a major consideration in temporary pacemakers.

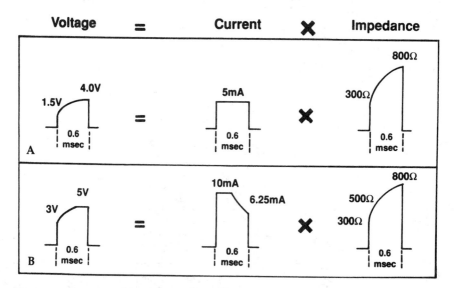

FIG. 3-4. Constant-current voltage-limited pacemaker spike. **A:** An idealized constant-current pacemaker with a 5-V battery is set to operate at 5 mA. Over the impedance range shown, the pacemaker acts like a true constant-current source. **B:** The same 5-V pacemaker is set to oper-ate at 10 mA. Once the impedance reaches 500 Ω, the pacemaker is using the entire 5-V bat-tery energy and cannot raise the voltage any higher; from that point on, it acts like a constant-voltage pacemaker.

Determination of Threshold

The threshold in cardiac pacing is the minimal electric stimulus required to cause cardiac muscle contraction. Having made that general statement, an accurate description of threshold is more complex.

Voltage and Current Threshold

Voltage threshold is the most commonly used measurement of pacing threshold. The pacing wire is placed in contact with the myocardium and connected to a commercially available pacing system analyzer that provides a constant-voltage power source. A specific pulse width is set (usually the pulse width of the permanent pacemaker to be used, such as 0.5 or 0.6 msec), and the rate of the pacemaker is set high enough to override the patient's intrinsic heart rate. The voltage is set high enough to stimulate the heart and then turned down until capture is lost (i.e., until the voltage is too low to stimulate the heart). The lowest voltage that stimulates the heart is the voltage threshold for that given pulse width. The current also can be measured in a similar manner to determine its threshold. There are two types of analyzers: one measures voltage and current at the beginning of the pacemaker spike, and the other measures voltage and current at the middle of the pacemaker spike. Thus, slightly different values may be found for the same patient.

In determining threshold, both the voltage and current thresholds should be measured, and the impedance of the pacing system should be calculated. Because the permanent pacemaker has a battery with limited voltage, the voltage threshold is the most clinically useful to report. For example, if a patient's myocardium has a chronic high threshold, and a special high-output 8-V pacing generator is being considered, then knowing the voltage threshold is essential. It would have to be below 8 V and preferably no higher than 5 V so that a 3-V safety margin would exist. Measuring the current threshold alone would not be helpful in this instance. Table 3-1 gives the usually obtainable and acceptable acute (at initial implant) and chronic thresholds and sensing values. Note that the maximum acceptable acute threshold at implant provides a safety margin to allow for the expected chronic threshold rise as well as sudden changes (such as higher threshold during sleep).

Pacemaker threshold should not be determined with a constant-current temporary pacemaker that does not give voltage and impedance information. The reason is that if the impedance of the pacing system is unexpectedly high, such as might occur with a partial lead fracture, a temporary constant-current pacing generator with a 15-V battery might give an acceptable current threshold value and not demonstrate the high-voltage threshold. The following example should clarify this point. If a patient had a current threshold of 2 mA and if a wire with an unusually high impedance of 5,000 Ω (because of a partial fracture) were in place, then a current setting of 2 mA on the temporary pacemaker would capture the heart. This is true because, according to Ohm's law ($V = iR$), 10 V is required

TABLE 3-1. *Threshold and sensing values for initial implant and generator change*[a]

I. Acute measurements (measured at a pulse width of 0.5 msec)
A. Threshold
1. Voltage: <1.0 V and preferably <-0.5 V (consider repositioning if initial threshold near 1.0 V)
2. Current: <1.5 mA
3. Impedance: approximately 400–1200 Ω
B. Sensing
1. R wave: >5 mV (peak to peak)
2. P wave: >2.0 and preferably >2.5–3.0 mV
II. Chronic measurements (measured at a pulse width of 0.5 msec)
A. Threshold
1. Voltage: <3.0 V
2. Current: <6 mA
3. Impedance: usually 500 Ω or so (if impedance very low, suspect insulation break; if impedance very high, suspect poor connection or lead fracture)
B. Sensing
1. R wave: >4 or 5 mV
2. P wave: >1.5, preferably 2.0–3.0 mV

[a]These are rough guidelines only. Patients with unusual threshold or sensing values need to be managed on an individual basis depending on the clinical situation. Atrial threshold and sensing values are less well established than those for ventricular pacing.

to generate the current through the high resistance, and the temporary pacemaker can generate up to 15 V. A permanent pacemaker, however, has only a 5-V battery and, again according to Ohm's law, could deliver only 1 mA of current through 5,000 Ω, which would be insufficient to stimulate the heart.

Energy threshold is another, but seldom used, measurement of threshold. It is the product of voltage, current, and pulse duration at threshold. It gives the total picture of energy required for depolarization and usually is expressed in microjoules.

Strength–Duration Curve

Another major determinant of threshold is the pulse width or pulse duration of the pacing spike. The relationship between pulse width and voltage threshold is important; the narrower the pulse width, the greater the voltage required to stimulate the heart. Most new permanent pacemakers allow pulse width to be programmed noninvasively. Figure 3-5 shows a strength–duration curve that is a plot of a hypothetical voltage stimulation threshold against pulse width. (As discussed in the following, threshold rises with time.) It is evident from the shape of the curve that increasing the pulse width to greater than 2.0 msec does little to improve voltage threshold. Although wider pulse widths up to 2.0 msec provide a lower voltage threshold, they also expend more electrons per pacemaker spike and cause the battery to discharge more rapidly. Therefore, most programmable permanent pacemakers have a pulse width range of approximately 0.1 to 2.0 msec, and a typical pulse width setting is 0.6 msec.

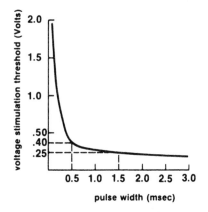

FIG. 3-5. Strength-duration curve. In this particular graph, the strength-duration curve of a newly implanted pacing electrode (acute threshold) is shown. At a pulse width of 0.5 msec, approximately 0.4 V is required to stimulate the heart. If the pulse width is increased to 1.5 msec, only 0.25 V or so are required to stimulate the heart. Only points above or on the curved line will cause cardiac stimulation.

Importance of Impedance in the System

The impedance in the wire should be extremely low, which is easily achieved with metal alloys that are extremely conductive. A high impedance in the wire or fracture would lead to a high resistance, which just would cause heat in the wire and be of no value in pacing. On the other hand, the impedance in the biological interface with the electrode tip actually may be beneficial if it is not too low. An average impedance in the system would be about 500 Ω; with only minimal impedance or resistance coming from the wire itself, most of that is because of the resistance as the electricity leaves the metal and enters the body (electrolyte solution) and then reenters metal to complete the circuit. A quite low impedance leads to a high current for every paced beat, and more electrons are expended per paced beat because of the low impedance. An extremely high impedance would make it impossible to pace, but a moderately high impedance with a good threshold (and low polarization with good sensing) actually leads to an ideal situation in which the heart is easily paced with a minimum number of electrons (i.e., less battery drain).

Threshold Changes

The threshold for a given patient does not remain static. Rapid changes can occur: Exercise or the pain and anxiety related to pacemaker insertion can increase levels of circulating catecholamines, causing lower thresholds; sleep can decrease catecholamine levels and raise thresholds.

Time produces a clinically more important change in threshold. A pacemaker wire usually has its lowest threshold (*acute threshold*) at the time of implantation. Over a period of 2 to 6 weeks, the threshold rises to its highest level at approximately three or four times the acute level and then falls to a chronic threshold that is usually stable at approximately two or three times the acute level (Fig. 3-6).

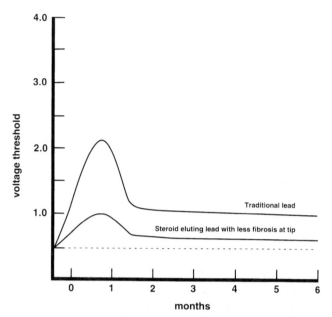

FIG. 3-6. Change in threshold. In this example, the acute threshold was 0.8 V and increased to 3.0 V shortly after implantation. After 3 or 4 months, the threshold stabilized at 2.0 V. All patients differ, but this graph shows a fairly typical change from acute to chronic threshold. The lower dotted line indicates lower thresholds in a more modern lead. This may be a porous tip or steroid-eluting lead, which usually results in lower thresholds.

    A simple and reasonably accurate way to conceptualize these changes is to think of the electrode tip as becoming larger with time. As we noted in Chapter 2, a large electrode tip produces less current density during the pacing spike, and therefore that current is less effective in stimulating the heart. The explanation of threshold change is shown in Figure 3-7. When first implanted, the electrode tip is in direct contact with excitable myocardium, and the threshold is at its lowest. After 3 weeks, edema and inflammation separate the metal tip from the myocardium. The electric charge is dispersed before reaching the myocardium, and the threshold is at its highest. After 6 months, the inflammation has died down, the tip is surrounded by fibrous tissue, and even though the threshold is still higher than at implant, it is lower than at 3 weeks because the electric charge is now less dispersed.

    One frequent misconception is that the threshold changes because the buildup of fibrous tissue increases impedance. In fact, the impedance remains unchanged. As far as the electricity is concerned, the fibrous tissue at the pacemaker tip is simply an electrolyte solution that conducts electricity as well as blood or muscle.

    In a small percentage of patients, the amount of fibrous tissue at the electrode tip may increase gradually. The chronic threshold will continue to rise and may become too high for a standard 5-V pacemaker to capture the heart.

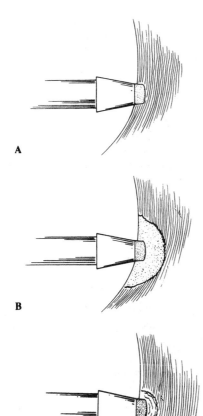

FIG. 3-7. Mechanism of change in threshold. **A:** Acute threshold of 0.5 V at implantation. The metal electrode tip is in direct contact with the myocardium. **B:** Peak threshold of 3.0 V at 3 weeks. Inflammatory cells separate the electrode and the excitable myocardium and disperse the pacing charge before it reaches the myocardium. **C:** Stable chronic threshold of 2.0 V at 6 months. A small, stable fibrous capsule has formed around the electrode tip. Steroid-eluting electrodes have been developed to reduce the transient acute rise in threshold.

Sensing

All modern pacemakers are designed to sense the patient's intrinsic heartbeat. In sensing, the principles of an electric circuit still apply, but the power source generating the current is the heart itself. As the heart muscle depolarizes, a potential difference is created between the tip and band electrodes of the bipolar wire or between the tip and the metal plate on the pacemaker wall in the unipolar wire. The pacemaker senses this difference as a weak electric signal. Impedance is associated with sensing and involves the impedance of the wires and electrolyte solution (i.e., the body) as well as polarization resistance; it is termed *source impedance* to differentiate it from the impedance occurring during the pacing spike.

The most commonly sensed cardiac event is ventricular depolarization resulting in the QRS complex. The shape of the QRS complex seen by the cardiac pacemaker has no relation to the shape of the QRS complex as seen on the surface electrocardiogram (ECG). The pacemaker sees an electrogram recorded directly from the endocardium of the heart. P-wave sensing has become more important with the increased use of dual-chamber pacemakers. The P wave, of course, has a lower amplitude and lower slew rate (see page 58) than the QRS complex, and so sensing problems are more common. With exercise, the P wave may diminish, and sensing may become more difficult.

Figure 3-8 shows electrograms taken at the time of implantation and approximately 1 year after implantation. The initial electrogram (acute) has ST segment elevation as a result of localized myocardial trauma where the electrode tip abuts the myocardium. Over a period of weeks or months, this acute electrogram becomes a chronic electrogram, with no ST segment elevation and a somewhat lower amplitude. Sensed electrograms can be recorded at the time of pacemaker implantation or at the time of battery change using the ECG connections shown in Figure 3-9.

Any QRS signal can be analyzed as the sum of an infinite number of sine waves. A simple example of this concept is shown in Fig. 3-10. The geometric figure on the left represents a QRS complex and can be approximated by summing large numbers of sine waves. The five largest of these pure frequencies are shown in the center, and on the right is the figure produced by summing the five waves. As greater numbers of smaller sine waves are added, the original figure is approximated more closely. This principle was investigated by Fourier, a French mathematician, and the set of pure frequencies representing the figure is called a *Fourier series*. In some pacemakers, the signal the pacemaker senses is actually the frequency of the sine waves inherent in the QRS signal. An analogy may clarify this concept. At a symphony, a single complex waveform strikes the listener's ear, but the notes of the individual instruments are heard because the pure frequencies can be separated from the complex waveform by the inner ear. (If this concept remains confusing, it can be ignored because an understanding of it is not necessary to practice clinically; it is presented mainly to make some of the more advanced studies on pacing accessible to the reader.) The clinician is not easily able to generate a Fourier series for the sensed electrogram, but two

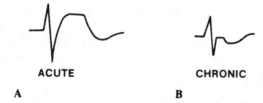

ACUTE   CHRONIC

A   B

FIG. 3-8. Intracardiac electrogram. **A:** Electrogram at the time of implantation with ST segment elevation. **B:** Chronic electrogram with no ST segment elevation and slightly lower amplitude.

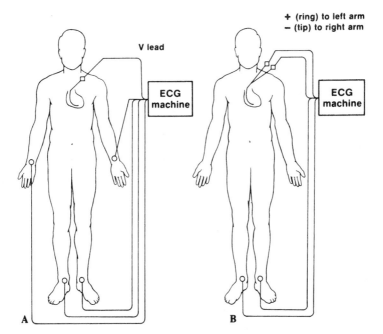

FIG. 3-9. Recording an electrogram. **A:** The unipolar connection required to record an electrogram from a unipolar electrode. The limb leads are put on the patient as usual, the electrode is connected to the V lead with a sterile clip, and the electrogram is recorded. **B:** For a bipolar electrode, the leg leads are put on the patient, but the left arm lead is connected to the positive (ring) electrode, and the right arm lead is connected to the negative (tip) electrode. Equipment must be properly grounded to prevent leakage of current to the heart that might cause ventricular arrhythmias.

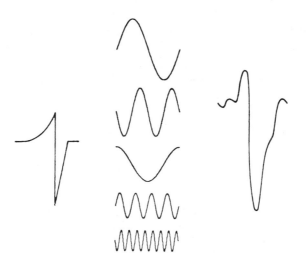

FIG. 3-10. QRS sensing. A hypothetical QRS complex sensed by the pacemaker appears on the left. In the center are the five largest pure frequencies inherent in the QRS complex. Summing of the five frequencies to approximate the QRS complex appears on the right. As larger numbers of smaller-amplitude and higher-frequency sine waves are added together, the QRS complex is approximated more closely. The pacemaker senses the largest pure frequencies inherent in the QRS complex.

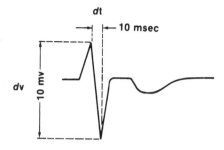

FIG. 3-11. Amplitude and slew rate. The amplitude of the electrogram in this example is 10 mV. The slew rate of the most rapidly moving portion of the QRS complex (the values shown by the dotted line) is 0.01 V/0.01 second, or 1 V per second.

useful measurements, amplitude and slew rate, can be obtained to estimate whether an electrogram falls within the sensing range of a pacemaker.

The amplitude of the electrogram is simply the total height (both positive and negative deflection) in millivolts of the QRS complex. In general, the greater the amplitude, the more likely it is that the QRS signal will be used. Slew rate is the rate of change in voltage in an electrogram. Mathematically, this is represented by dv/dt. Figure 3-11 demonstrates the concept of slew rate and amplitude. In general, the greater the slew rate of an electrogram, the more likely it is to be sensed.

In clinical practice, the slew rate rarely is measured; in fact, simply measuring the amplitude of the sensed QRS complex is almost always sufficient to estimate whether a QRS complex is likely to be sensed. Most pacemaker manufacturers describe the sensitivity of the pacemakers in millivolts (i.e., QRS height) for simplicity. New pacing system analyzers can measure slew rate of the sensed electrogram automatically. As discussed in the preceding, polarization resistance is decreased if the surface area of the metal in contact with the electrolyte is increased. Thus, sensing is better with a large electrode tip than with a small tip. On the other hand, stimulation threshold is lowered with the smaller electrode tip because the current density is greater. One type of electrode developed in an attempt to combine a large surface area for better sensing with a high charge concentration for lower threshold pacing is the porous tip electrode shown in Fig. 3-12.

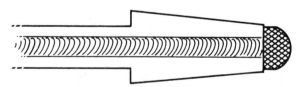

FIG. 3-12. Porous tip electrode. The diameter of the exposed metal tip is small to produce higher current density and better pacing thresholds. The tip is made of a porous metal mesh (or carbon material) so that the area of metal in contact with the electrolyte solution is large, thereby lowering polarization resistance and increasing the ability of the pacemaker to sense. This is shown partly to emphasize the concepts of current density and polarization resistance.

TEMPORARY PACING APPLICATIONS

Most of the electrophysiology pertinent to temporary pacing has been discussed in this chapter, and we will summarize briefly. Temporary pacemakers almost always have constant-current circuitry. Because a typical temporary generator supplies approximately 15 V, the current can be kept truly constant over a relatively high range of impedance compared with permanent constant-current pacemakers that supply a maximum of 5 V. It is important that temporary pacemakers not be used to determine the threshold for permanent pacemakers.

The higher voltage of the temporary pacemaker battery allows pacing even at moderately high thresholds; so, although obtaining the lowest possible threshold is important with a temporary pacemaker, the system is more forgiving should a higher threshold be encountered.

The pulse width of temporary pacemakers is fixed at approximately 1.8 msec. Although this wide pulse width consumes more energy, conservation of battery life is not a consideration in temporary pacemakers. Thus, a broad pulse width that gives the lowest threshold is used; this feature need not be programmable. As stated previously, little improvement in threshold occurs if the pulse width is greater than approximately 0.6 msec, and essentially no improvement occurs with pulse widths greater than about 1.8 msec.

REFERENCES

Baker RG Jr, Falkenberg EN. Bipolar versus unipolar issues in DDD pacing (Part II). *Pacing Clin Electrophysiol* 1984;7:1178.

Barold SS, Ong LS, Heinle RA. Stimulation and sensing thresholds for cardiac pacing: electrophysiologic and technical aspects. *Prog Cardiovasc Dis* 1981;24:1.

Breivik K, Ohm O-J, Engedal H. Long-term comparison of unipolar and bipolar pacing and sensing, using a new multiprogrammable pacemaker system (Part I). *Pacing Clin Electrophysiol* 1983;6:592.

Chew P, Bush D, Engel B, Talan M, Abell R. Overnight heart rate and cardiac function in patients with dual chamber pacemakers. *Pacing Clin Electrophysiol* 1996;19:822.

Clarke M, Liu B, Schuller H, et al. Automatic adjustment of pacemaker stimulation output correlated with continuously monitored capture thresholds: a multicenter study. *Pacing Clin Electrophysiol* 1998;21:1567.

Cornacchia D, Fabbri M, Maresta A, et al. Effect of steroid eluting versus conventional electrodes on propafenone induced rise in chronic ventricular pacing threshold. *Pacing Clin Electrophysiol* 1993;16:2279.

Furman S, Garvey J, Hurzeler P. Pulse duration variation and electrode size as factors in pacemaker longevity. *J Thorac Cardiovasc Surg* 1975;69:382.

Furman S, Parker B, Escher DJW, Solomon N. Endocardial threshold of cardiac response as a function of electrode surface area. *J Surg Res* 1968;8:161.

Hill WE, Murray A, Bourke JP, et al. Minimum energy for cardiac pacing. *Clin Phys Physiol Meas* 1988;9:41.

Klein HH, Steinberger J, Knake W. Stimulation characteristics of a steroid-eluting electrode compared with three conventional electrodes. *Pacing Clin Electrophysiol* 1990;13:134.

Kruse IM. Long-term performance of endocardial leads with steroid-eluting electrodes (Part II). *Pacing Clin Electrophysiol* 1986;9:1217.

Kulakowski P, Malik M, Odemuyiwa O, et al. Frequency versus time domain analysis of the signal-averaged electrocardiogram: reproducibility of the spectral turbulence analysis (Part I). *Pacing Clin Electrophysiol* 1993;16:1027.

Mond H, Stokes K, Helland J, et al. The porous titanium steroid eluting electrode: a double blind study assessing the stimulation threshold effects of steroid. *Pacing Clin Electrophysiol* 1988;11:214.

Moracchini P, Cornacchia D, Bernasconi M, et al. High impedence low energy pacing leads: long-term results with a very small surface area steroid-eluting lead compared to three conventional electrodes. *Pacing Clin Electrophysiol* 1999;22:326.

Preston TA, Judge RD. Alteration of pacemaker threshold by drug and physiological factors. *Ann NY Acad Sci* 1969;167:686.

Schuchert A, Hopf M, Kuck KH, Bleifeld W. Chronic ventricular electrograms: do steroid-eluting leads differ from conventional leads (Part II)? *Pacing Clin Electrophysiol* 1990;13:1879.

Sermasi S, Marconi M, Libero L, et al. Italian experience with autocapture in conjunction with a membrane lead (Part II). *Pacing Clin Electrophysiol* 1996;19:1799.

Shepard R, Kim J, Colvin E, Slabaugh J, Epstein A, Bargeron L. Pacing threshold spikes months and years after implant (Part II). *Pacing Clin Electrophysiol* 1991;14:1835.

4

Programmability and Specialized Circuits

PERMANENT PACEMAKER PROGRAMMABILITY

Programmability often allows for noninvasive correction of pacemaker malfunction. We emphasize, however, that inappropriate use of external programming may be dangerous. Before a pacing problem is corrected with external programming, the problem must be appropriately diagnosed and the clinical status of the patient, especially the degree of the patient's pacemaker dependency and the safety margin left after programming, must be considered.

Methods of External Programming

Early in the development of permanent pacemakers, the advantage of being able to change the rate of firing of the generator became obvious. One of the earliest efforts involved a screw on the generator that, when turned, would change the pacing rate. This method required making a skin incision and using a sterile screwdriver. Advances in technology now allow noninvasive programming of several pacemaker functions, including rate. To program a pacemaker externally, a signal, usually pulsed magnetic fields or a radiofrequency signal, is sent through the patient's skin and received by the generator. If a pulsed magnetic field is transmitted, it can influence a small, thin, flat piece of metal called a *reed switch* to bend slightly, touch another metal terminal, and thus complete an electrical circuit. The pacemaker must be protected against accidental or phantom programming resulting from bombardment of the pacemaker by environmental electromagnetic waves. Usually this protection requires that a very specific code be sensed by the pacemaker before it will respond to programming.

Rate Programmability

The pacemaker function most commonly programmed is *rate*. A typical programmable range is 30 to 120 bpm, and most pacemakers are preset by the manufacturer at approximately 70 bpm. Many studies have attempted to determine the pacemaker rate that optimizes cardiac output, and, in general, it has been found that cardiac output varies little over a fairly wide range of paced rates, even when an atrial pacemaker is used. The increase in cardiac output that occurs normally with exercise involves not only an increase in heart rate but also peripheral vasodilatation in areas of increased metabolic activity and an increase in cardiac contractility. Simply increasing the rate of the pacemaker does not duplicate these complex physiologic events. In some individual patients and in some clinical situations, however, an increase in pacemaker rate does increase cardiac output. For example, a pacemaker-dependent patient who is metabolically unstable after surgery may benefit from a faster-paced rate. If the clinical situation is critical, this could even be determined by use of thermodilution cardiac outputs. Rate programmability allows for flexibility in these instances. Another reason for increasing rate is to overdrive cardiac arrhythmias.

Pacemaker rate is decreased most commonly to allow the emergence of the patient's spontaneous rhythm. Many patients with sinus bradycardia feel better with the atrial "kick" that increases cardiac output than with a ventricularly paced rhythm at a faster rate. In addition, this slowing of the paced rate preserves battery life. Decreasing the paced rate is used less commonly to determine the patient's underlying rhythm or to observe the patient's intrinsic electrocardiogram (ECG) to evaluate a possible myocardial infarction or assess drug effects on ECG intervals. Table 4-1 summarizes the uses of rate programmability.

Pulse-width Programmability

As discussed in Chapter 3, the width or duration of the pacemaker spike is of considerable clinical importance, even though it cannot be measured on a standard 12-lead ECG. Either an oscilloscope or a hand-held, commercially available pulse width measuring device can be used to determine the exact time duration of the pacemaker impulse.

Widening the pulse width improves the ability of the pacemaker to stimulate the heart, but as predicted by the strength–duration curve, this improvement is

---

TABLE 4-1. *Uses of rate programmability*

1. Optimizing cardiac output in the unusual patient who requires a specific rate for best cardiac output and in unusual clinical situations such as in a pacemaker-dependent patient who is medically unstable with a low cardiac output
2. Overdrive suppression of arrhythmias
3. Increasing battery longevity by decreasing rate
4. Increasing the amount of time a patient is in sinus rhythm (with augmented cardiac output due to the atrial kick) by decreasing rate
5. Evaluation of intrinsic ECG to assess:
   a. Underlying rhythm
   b. Myocardial infarction
   c. Drug effect on the ECG
   d. Effect of a metabolic abnormality on the ECG

ECG, electrocardiogram.

only a modest one at greater widths. An example of widening the pulse width to allow capture of the heart rate is shown in Figure 4-1. At the time of pacemaker implantation, the patient had a good acute threshold of 0.6 V when the pulse width was 0.6 msec; however, after 4 weeks, the threshold rose to approximately 5 V with a pulse width of 0.6 msec, and the patient was intermittently losing capture. Slight widening of the pulse width caused consistent capture. To allow a reasonable safety factor, the pulse width in the example was left at 1.8 msec.

We are using an example in which capture is improved, but often the strength-duration curve is so flat beyond 0.5 msec that a widened pulse width may not improve capture safely and effectively. Also, we are assuming that no other evidence of pacemaker malfunction, such as electrode displacement, is present and that the patient is not so pacemaker dependent that any further threshold rise causing transient loss of capture would be a risk to the patient. Another approach to the problem would be to raise the voltage of the pacemaker above 5 V, but this is not technically possible with all pacing devices.

If the clinician believes that widening the pulse width is reasonably safe in such a situation, then doing so may save the patient a surgical procedure; in fact, the threshold may improve with time. The tradeoff with the widened pulse width is a shorter battery life, but with the long-lived lithium batteries, battery life often is not a major consideration. Some companies provide a chart listing estimated battery life in relation to pulse width for a given paced rate. The relationship between pulse width and battery depletion is not linear: Doubling the pulse width shortens battery life by less than half. This happens because the first half of the pacemaker spike generates more current than the second half (see Fig. 3-3).

Another use of programming pulse width is to preserve battery life. In the example depicted in Figure 4-2, a patient has a low chronic threshold of 5 V at 0.1-msec pulse width. Because the battery is fixed at 5 V, energy is wasted. By narrowing the pulse width from the usual 0.5 msec to 0.3 msec, energy is preserved (i.e., fewer electrons are expended per pacing spike, and therefore battery life is prolonged), and a reasonable safety margin still exists. The patient still

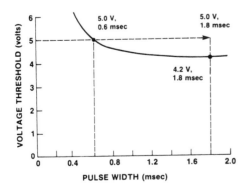

FIG. 4-1. Widening pulse width to maintain capture. In this example, the patient's threshold rose to 5 V when the pacer spike was at 0.6 msec. By increasing the duration of the pacer spike to 1.8 msec, capture can now occur at approximately 4.2 V. Because this particular pacemaker generates only 5 V, the safety margin may not be adequate for all patients.

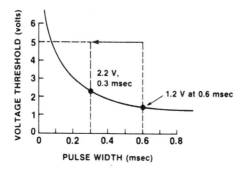

FIG. 4-2. Narrowing pulse width to preserve battery life. In this example, the patient has a low chronic threshold of 1.2 V at 0.6-msec pulse width. Because the battery is fixed at 5 V, energy is wasted. By narrowing the pulse width to 0.3 msec, energy is preserved and a reasonable safety margin still exists.

should be monitored periodically to ensure that the threshold is not rising. Another approach to preserving battery life in this situation would be to lower voltage if voltage were programmable. (Although voltage cannot be raised easily, it can be lowered easily in most pacemakers.)

Programming pulse width can be used to estimate threshold. Figures 4-1 and 4-2 are drawn as if we knew the shape of the strength–duration curve in both patients; this is done for the sake of explaining concepts. In practice, however, the exact shape of the strength–duration curve in an individual patient often is unknown. Therefore, we can obtain an estimate of the threshold as determined by pulse width at a fixed voltage (i.e., one point on the strength-duration curve) by narrowing pulse width until capture is lost. This information is sometimes clinically useful. With newer units that feature voltage programmability, additional points on the strength–duration curve can be obtained.

Narrowing pulse width also can be used to reduce annoying electric complications of pacing, such as pectoral muscle twitching or diaphragmatic stimulation, that occur in an occasional patient, although this approach is usually not successful; lowering voltage is a better approach. Before programming is done, the pacing system should be checked to ensure that no malfunction requiring another method of correction is causing the difficulty. Table 4-2 summarizes the use of pulse width programmability.

TABLE 4-2. *Uses of pulse width programmability*

1. Increase pulse width to capture the heart in a patient with high threshold[a]
2. Narrow pulse width to reduce annoying electrical side effects of pacing such as pectoral muscle or diaphragmatic stimulation (although this usually is an unsuccessful maneuver)
3. Narrow pulse width to preserve battery life
4. Assess threshold (as determined by pulse width at a fixed voltage)

[a]Before using pulse width programming to troubleshoot these problems, the entire pacemaker system should be evaluated as well as the clinical status of the patient to ensure that another mode of therapy such as electrode revision of generator change would not be more appropriate. Also, a reasonable safety margin must be left in the system for chronic and acute rises in threshold.

Voltage Programmability

Some pacemakers offer multiple settings that can be externally programmed. Some allow programming above 5 V, but most commercially available pacemakers at present can be programmed only to lower voltage settings. Increasing voltage may maintain capture in a patient with a poor threshold but at the expense of more rapid battery depletion. High-voltage units that consist of two lithium iodine batteries in series are available.

Being able to lower the voltage setting by programming allows conservation of battery life, as demonstrated in Fig. 4-3. In this example, the patient has an unusually low chronic threshold of 1.3 V at 0.6-msec pulse width. By leaving the voltage at 2.5 V and pulse width at 0.6 msec, fewer electrons are used per paced beat, and battery life is preserved. It should be emphasized that this approach is useful only if the chronic threshold is low and if battery life is a significant clinical consideration in the patient. Another approach to this patient would be to narrow pulse width.

The voltage programmability along with pulse width programmability also can be used to determine threshold noninvasively. These uses are listed in Table 4-3.

Sensitivity Circuit and Programmability

In Chapter 3, we discussed that the pacemaker senses the intrinsic frequency of the QRS complex, but clinically we estimate whether a QRS complex will be sensed by measuring its total height (positive and negative deflection) and, less commonly, the slew rate. The QRS complex generates a weak current in the pacing system, and this signal then is amplified. The amplification requires a modest amount of battery energy but not nearly as much as is required for pacing. Many signals unrelated to the QRS complex, such as current due to pectoral muscle activity or external electromagnetic interference, cause weak currents in pacing systems. To reduce the possibility that these currents will be inappropri-

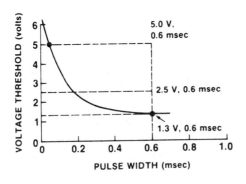

FIG. 4-3. Lowering voltage to prolong battery life. This patient's chronic threshold is unusually low and stable, and not all 5 V are required to pace the patient at a pulse width of 0.6 msec. The low threshold is demonstrated by programming the voltage to 1.3 V and observing that capture is still maintained. By leaving the voltage at 2.5 V, a safety margin is established and battery life is conserved.

TABLE 4-3. *Uses of voltage programmability*

---

1. Decrease voltage to preserve battery life (if clinically indicated and if chronic voltage threshold is low and stable)
2. Increase voltage to maintain capture in a patient with a high threshold
3. Use in conjunction with pulse width programmability to determine pacing threshold noninvasively (points on the strength-duration curve can be obtained)
4. Lower voltage to reduce annoying electrical side effects of pacing such as pectoral muscle or diaphragmatic stimulation (sometimes a successful maneuver)

---

ately sensed as QRS complexes, two additional components are added to the sensing circuit. One is a level detector to prevent low-level electrical noise from being sensed. The other is a bandpass filter to help eliminate stronger signals that are of a different frequency than those associated with the QRS complex. A schematic diagram of the sensing circuit is shown in Figure 4-4, and the principle of the bandpass filter is shown in Figure 4-5.

The programmable feature of the sensing circuit is usually the level detector. By causing the level detector to block weaker signals, the sensitivity of the pacemaker is lessened. Such a programming change could be used to prevent inappropriate sensing of a T wave, after-potential, or pectoral muscle activity (one hopes without loss of the intrinsic QRS signal), for example. Alternately, by causing the level detector to pass on weaker signals, the sensitivity of the pacemaker can be increased. The latter programming change could be used to allow sensing of unusually weak QRS signals, for example, a signal that was initially weak at the time of lead placement and became weaker with the decrease in amplitude and slew rate that normally occurs over time (due to fibrosis at the tip of the electrode).

Noise-sensing Circuit

Although a noise-sensing circuit is not programmable, we mention it here because it relates to sensing. The level detector and bandpass filter of the sensing circuit prevent many inappropriate signals from being sensed, but they are not infallible, especially when signals from the environment are strong. Therefore, many pacemakers have additional protection against electromagnetic interference (EMI) because mistaking EMI for a QRS signal will cause the pacemaker to stop firing.

One method of protecting against EMI is to have a noise-sampling period in each cycle that listens for several repetitions of a signal within a few milliseconds. Obviously, only one QRS signal can occur in a few milliseconds; if several signals are received, the pacemaker is programmed to fire in an asynchronous mode regardless of the patient's intrinsic heart rate. Although this program could cause the pacemaker to fire even if the patient's rate was faster than the paced rate, this disadvantage is outweighed by the advantage of preventing EMI from

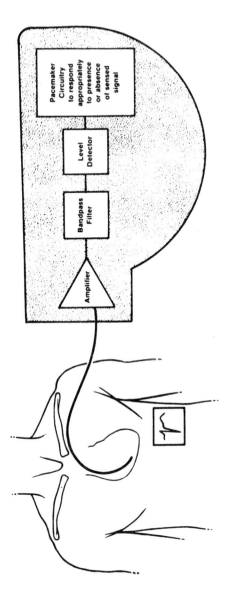

FIG. 4-4. Sensing circuit. The amplifier, which uses a small amount of current to increase the weak sensed QRS signal (or in an atrial pacer, the P-wave signal), the bandpass filter, and the level detector in a sensing circuit are demonstrated. External programming allows the level detector setting to be changed so that more signals can be detected or blocked, depending on whether sensitivity is to be increased or decreased.

shutting off a pacemaker in a pacemaker-dependent patient. Thus, in diagnosing the cause of inappropriate sensing by a pacemaker, the presence of EMI must be considered if the pacemaker contains a noise-sensing circuit. In another method of protecting against EMI, the pacemaker constantly samples and disregards background noise so that only the single, prominent QRS signal is detected.

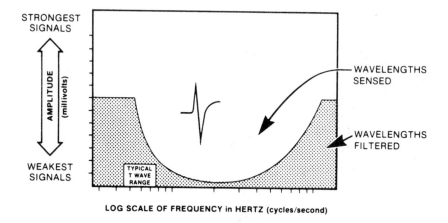

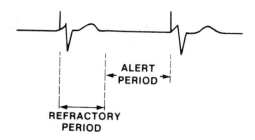

FIG. 4-5. Bandpass filter. The shaded area is filtered out by the bandpass filter, and only frequencies commonly associated with the QRS complex are allowed to pass through the sensing circuit.

Refractory Period Programmability

All pacemakers' timing circuitry includes a method of turning off the sensing ability for a brief period after either a sensed QRS signal or a pacemaker spike (or at least ignoring any sensed signals during this time). This refractory period is depicted in Figure 4-6. The advantage of a refractory period is that it does not

FIG. 4-6. Refractory period after paced beat. During the refractory period, the sensing circuit of the pacemaker is turned off so that it will not inappropriately sense the QRS or the T wave of any beat or the after-potential of a paced beat. In some models, sensing may occur during the refractory period, but the pacemaker does not reset its timing cycle during the refractory period. The time of the refractory period varies among manufacturers and is externally programmable in some. In some pacemakers, the refractory period after a paced beat is longer than after a sensed beat.

allow the pacemaker to sense either the T wave of the preceding QRS complex or the pacemaker after-potential, which is residual electric activity occurring after a paced beat. Although the bandpass filter and level detector should prevent such inappropriate sensing, they are not foolproof. The only disadvantage of such a circuit is that early premature ventricular contractions (PVCs) may not be sensed, but the advantage of eliminating a common source of inappropriate sensing is more important. The physician who sees an unsensed early PVC on a pacemaker ECG must know whether the pacemaker has a refractory period and what that period is to know whether the pacemaker is responding appropriately to the PVC. Note that, in pacing, the term *refractory period* is used somewhat differently than it is in electrophysiology.

The refractory period can be lengthened to eliminate inappropriate sensing of a QRS signal, T wave, or after-potential. An example of lengthening the refractory period is shown in Figure 4-7. A demand atrial pacemaker has been placed and is programmed to fire at a rate of 72 bpm. The QRS of the paced beat falls outside the refractory period and is sensed by the pacemaker, which causes the pacemaker to reset its timing cycle and therefore fire at a rate slower than 72 bpm. By lengthening the refractory period, the QRS is no longer sensed and the pacemaker fires at an appropriate rate of 72 bpm. The refractory period rarely needs to be shortened. One example is shown in Fig. 4-8, in which nonsensing of a PVC is prevented.

As discussed in Chapter 5, the atrial refractory period in a dual-chamber pacemaker can be lengthened in some instances to avoid an endless loop pacemaker-mediated arrhythmia. Table 4-4 summarizes the uses of refractory period programmability.

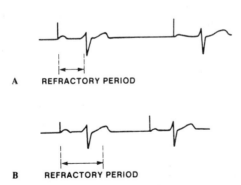

A   **REFRACTORY PERIOD**

B   **REFRACTORY PERIOD**

FIG. 4-7. Refractory period lengthening in an atrial pacemaker. **A:** The QRS complex falls outside the refractory period of the pacemaker and is sensed by the pacemaker, which causes the timing cycle to reset and results in a rate slower than the programmed rate. **B:** The refractory period has been extended beyond the QRS complex, and the pacemaker now fires at the programmed rate.

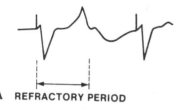

A   **REFRACTORY PERIOD**

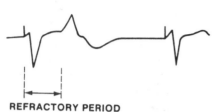

B   **REFRACTORY PERIOD**

FIG. 4-8. Refractory period shortening. **A:** The premature ventricular contraction (PVC) falls within the refractory period of the pacemaker and is not sensed. **B:** By shortening the refractory period, the PVC is sensed, the pacemaker timing cycle is reset, and more time is allowed for ventricular filling before the next paced beat. The pacer spike does not fall near the T wave of the PVC.

Hysteresis Programmability

Hysteresis, in pacing terminology, refers to the response pattern shown in Figure 4-9. In this example, the pacemaker does not begin firing until the patient's rate drops below 60 bpm; it then fires at a rate of 72 bpm. It will continue firing until one of the patient's intrinsic beats is sensed, and it will not fire again until the patient's rate drops below 60 bpm. Various escape intervals and pacing rates can be combined, but the escape interval is always greater than the interval between paced beats.

Hysteresis is potentially valuable in a patient who is often affected with sinus bradycardia and tolerates it well but requires a reasonably fast-paced rate to maintain adequate cardiac output during transient periods of asystole or during marked bradycardia when the pacemaker fires and atrial kick is lost. Besides leaving the patient in sinus rhythm for longer periods, hysteresis helps to preserve pacemaker battery life. Another obvious way to achieve the same result in our example is to leave the pacemaker set at 60 bpm. Assuming the patient tolerates a paced rate of 60 bpm and does not require a faster-paced rate to maintain adequate cardiac output (which most patients do not), programming the pacemaker to a lower rate is equally effective and simpler.

TABLE 4-4. *Uses of refractory period programmability*

---

1. Lengthen refractory period to correct inappropriate sensing of the preceding QRS complex, T wave, or after-potential of a paced beat (changing sensitivity may be another way to approach the problem)
2. Shorten refractory period to allow sensing of premature ventricular contractions not being sensed because they fall within the refractory period
3. Lengthen the atrial refractory period of a dual-chamber DDD or VDD pacemaker to avoid endless loop pacemaker-mediated arrhythmias (see Chapter 6)

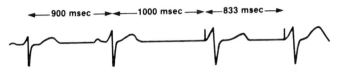

FIG. 4-9. In this example of a pacing unit with hysteresis, the pacemaker will not fire as long as the patient's intrinsic heart rate is greater than 60 bpm (RR interval of less than 1,000 msec). When the patient's rate slows to less than 60 beats, the pacemaker fires (escape interval of 1,000 msec), but it then fires at a rate of 72 bpm (RR interval of 833 msec) and continues to do so until it senses another beat, at which time the escape interval again will be 1,000 msec.

A relatively new use of hysteresis is in the patient with neurocardiogenic syncope (vasovagal syncope or hypersensitive carotid sinus syndrome) with a slow heart rate as well as a vasodepressor response. These patients have syncope or near syncope as a result of the combination of a drop in blood pressure and a slow heart rate. The drop in blood pressure cannot be altered with the pacemaker, but the slow heart rate can. Instead of having simple pacing [usually atrioventrivular (AV) sequential pacing], the pacemaker can be programmed to sense a sudden drop in slow heart rate and, when that occurs, pace quite rapidly for at least a brief period and then gradually decrease the rate. This requires a more complicated program in the pacemaker, but with today's technology that is relatively simple.

One potential problem with the use of hysteresis is that if the paced beat were to travel retrograde through the AV node and capture the atrium consistently, the patient would tend to be locked into the relatively rapid paced rate. Fortunately, this rarely occurs. The more common situation is for the atria to beat at their intrinsic rates without being depolarized by the ventricular paced beat, and once a single atrial beat captures the ventricle, the pacemaker is inhibited. The patient's own rhythm then resumes even though the patient's rate may be lower than the paced rate. Another problem with hysteresis is that it often confuses physicians.

Mode Programmability

Some pacemakers allow programmability into three pacing modes: ventricular demand, ventricular triggered, and asynchronous. This programmable feature is seldom used, but it has some advantages in that the ventricular triggered mode is more immune to EMI and the asynchronous mode is totally immune to EMI. The ability to switch to the asynchronous mode could be useful in a patient undergoing surgery that requires use of electrocautery. If a pacemaker were suspected of improperly sensing pectoral muscle stimulation or a T wave, programming to the ventricular triggered mode would cause a pacemaker spike to be placed on the sensed event, aiding in diagnosing the problem. The ventricular trigger spike is virtually never used nowadays. The same information can be obtained by more modern telemetry or marker channel devices that indicate what the pacemaker is sensing.

TEMPORARY PACEMAKER PROGRAMMABILITY

Rate Programmability

A typical pacing range for an external temporary pacemaker is 30 to 180 bpm, and the rate can be changed simply by turning a dial to the desired setting (Fig. 4-10). The uses of rate programmability in temporary pacing are identical to those of permanent pacing. The rapid temporary pacemaker rates are sometimes used to interrupt tachycardias.

Energy Output

Almost all external pacemakers are constant-current generators with a power source of approximately 15 V (a 9-V battery with a special circuit to raise the voltage). The energy output is measured in current (milliamperes, mA) and usually ranges from 0.1 to 20 mA (see Fig. 4-10). Because a typical acute threshold is lower than 1 or 2 mA and temporary pacemakers are not left in place long enough to warrant concern over chronic thresholds, the ability to raise energy output considerably allows maintenance of capture in patients in whom (a) low initial thresholds cannot be obtained, (b) threshold rises because of inflammation at the lead tip, or (c) poor lead position results in poor thresholds. If the current is very high, however, diaphragmatic or chest wall muscle stimulation may cause patient discomfort.

By turning down the current output until capture is lost, the threshold can easily be checked on a daily basis and, if indicated, the underlying rhythm can be determined. Underlying rhythm also can be checked by turning down the rate.

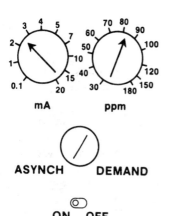

FIG. 4-10. Temporary pacemaker programmability. The three programmable functions of a temporary pacemaker are energy output (in milliamperes, mA), rate (in paced beats per minute, ppm), and sensitivity (either demand or asynchronous mode). (See text for details.)

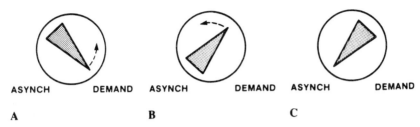

FIG. 4-11. Temporary pacemaker sensitivity settings. **A:** The pacemaker functions in the demand mode at maximum sensitivity. **B:** The pacemaker is still functioning in the demand mode, but sensitivity has been decreased. This setting would be useful if, for example, oversensing of a T wave were occurring. **C:** No sensing occurs.

Sensitivity

Most temporary pacemakers have a single dial to control sensitivity (Fig. 4-11; see also Fig. 4-10). When the dial is set on demand, the pacemaker is at maximum sensitivity. As the dial is turned toward asynchronous, the sensitivity decreases. Changing this setting may be useful in eliminating inappropriate sensing of the T wave. If the dial is turned completely to the asynchronous setting, no sensing occurs, and the pacemaker fires at the set rate regardless of the patient's own rhythm.

The pulse width is not programmable and is kept constant at approximately 1.8 msec, which is as wide as is practically useful. Narrower pulse widths are not required because battery longevity is not a consideration, and pulse widths greater than 1.8 msec do not improve the pacemaker's ability to capture the heart.

REFERENCES

Astrinsky EA, Furman S. Pacemaker output programming for maximum safety and maximum longevity. *Clin Prog Pacing Electrophysiol* 1983;1:51.

Frielingsdorf J, Gerber AE, Dur P, et al. Importance of an individually programmed atrioventricular delay at rest and on work capacity in patients with dual chamber pacemakers. *Pacing Clin Electrophysiol* 1994;17:37.

Gillis AM, Rothschild JM, Hillier K, et al. A randomized comparison of a bipolar steroid-eluting electrode and a bipolar microporous platinum electrode: implications for long-term programming (Part I). *Pacing Clin Electrophysiol* 1993;16:964.

Jones B, Kim J, Zhu Q, et al. Future of bradyarrhythmia therapy systems: automaticity. *Am J Cardiol* 1999;83:192D.

Saoudi N, Appl U, Anselme F, Voglimacci M, Cribier A. How smart should pacemakers be? *Am J Cardiol* 1999;83:180D.

Schoenfeld MH. A primer on pacemaker programmers. *Pacing Clin Electrophysiol* 1993;16:2044.

Stirbys P. A challenge: development of a universal programmer (Part I). *Pacing Clin Electrophysiol* 1993;16:693.

Wilson JH, Siegmund JB, Johnson R, et al. Pacing system analyzers: different systems-different results. *PACE* 1994;17:17.

5

Types of Pacemakers and Hemodynamics of Pacing

The use of pacemakers for antiarrhythmic therapy is a complex and frequently changing area of medicine. New antiarrhythmic drugs are under investigation, and new catheter-mediated techniques for cure of intractable arrhythmias have been developed. With the ever-increasing complexity of the advanced function pacemaker and the need for appropriate interpretation of complex pacemaker electrocardiograms (ECGs), pacing has evolved into a subspecialty within cardiology, alongside cardiac electrophysiology.

Historically, the implantation process was considered the most demanding aspect of pacemaking, but the procedure has been greatly simplified since the introduction of endocardial leads and the great reduction in size of the generators. Today, the appropriate selection of the device, programming, and troubleshooting for potential pacemaker dysfunction are considered the most difficult aspects and require additional skill and experience.

This chapter discusses the different types of pacemakers commonly used and the important aspects of hemodynamics of pacing and provides guidelines to aid in deciding which device is most appropriate for implantation.

PACEMAKER CODE

In 1974, the American Heart Association originally proposed the use of a three-letter code in describing the various types of pacemakers and their functions. Since then, the code was expanded to a five-letter code by the North American Society of Pacing and Electrophysiology (NASPE) and the British Pacing and Electrophysiology Group (BPEG). Thus, what was originally referred to as the ICHD (Inter-Society Commission for Heart Disease Resources) pacemaker code has been changed to the NBG code (combining NASPE and BPEG). The character positions in the code are labeled I through

V. The first three positions assume a fundamentally greater importance than the last two.

Position I refers to the chamber(s) being paced. The designation O refers to a situation in which bradycardia pacing is not an option of the device, such as in certain older model implantable cardioverter–defibrillators.

Position II refers to the chamber(s) being sensed. In the situations of single-chamber pacing or sensing, the designation *S* for positions I and II is available for the manufacturer to use in a generic manner because its application can be for either atrial or ventricular sites. The designation *O* refers to absent sensing (and thus refers to fixed, asynchronous pacing).

Position III refers to the device's response to sensing. *I* represents the inhibited mode, meaning that when the pacemaker senses an event, it will be inhibited from further pacing; this is the most common form of sensing. *T* indicates a triggered response. When the pacemaker senses an event, it will trigger the device to deliver a pacing stimulus. In single-chamber situations, the sensed event and triggered impulse occur within the same chamber. In a dual-chamber application, however, an atrial sensed event inhibits atrial stimulation and triggers the delivery of a ventricular stimulus with atrioventricular (AV) interval delay similar to that of a normal PR interval.

Position IV deals with programmability of rate modulation. *O* infers that none of the functions of the pacemaker can be altered using a programmer. *P* stands for simple programmability and means that only one or two features can be programmed. Usually, these are *rate* and *output*, but the code does not specify in greater detail. *M* refers to multiprogrammability, meaning that three or more features can be programmed. (Some of these features are discussed in Chapter 4.) *C* stands for "communicating" and indicates that the pacemaker has the capability of telemetry when used with the appropriate programmer. This usually refers to the ability to record real-time electrograms, the display of event markers (events sensed or paced), or the display of derived measurements such as lead impedance. *R* refers to rate modulation, in which a physiologic sensor is used to modify the rate of the pacemaker based on the patient's activity or metabolic need (see Chapter 7).

Position V is reserved for devices that have antitachycardia function. Terminatation of a tachycardia can be performed by the repetitive delivery of pacing stimuli (the letter *P* in the code) or by delivering a countershock (the letter *S* in the code). The code does not specify the particular regimen used in the pacing sequence or the output waveform or energy content of the countershock pulse.

From a practical point of view, only the first three letters are in common use, and an *R* is placed at the end if rate modulation is an option with the device. The NBG code is provided in Table 5-1.

TABLE 5-1. *The NASPE[a]/BPEG[b] (NBG[c]) generic pacemaker code*

Position	I	II	III	IV	V
Category	Chamber(s) paced:	Chamber(s) sensed:	Response to sensing:	Programmability, rate modulation:	Antitachyarrhythmia function(s):
	O = None	O = None	O = None	O = None	O = None
	A = Atrium	A = Atrium	T = Triggered	P = Simple programmable	P = Pacing (anti-tachyarrhythmia)
	V = Ventricle	V = Ventricle	I = Inhibited	M = Multiprogrammable	S = Shock
	D = Dual (A + V)	D = Dual (A + V)	D = Dual (T + I)	C = Communicating	S = Dual (P + S)
				R = Rate modulation	
Manufacturer's designation only	S = Single (A or V)	S = Single (A or V)			

[a]NASPE = North American Society for Pacing and Electrophysiology.
[b]BPEG = British Pacing and Electrophysiology Group.
[c]NBG = NASPE and British Group.

SINGLE-CHAMBER PERMANENT PACEMAKERS

From a practical standpoint, there are essentially only two forms of single-chamber pacing: VVI and AAI, with the former being the most common. Of course, rate modulation is an option for either chamber. AAI pacing is selected only for patients in whom the bradyarrhythmia is a sinus mechanism and AV block is not a problem. Such patients should not have chronic or intermittent atrial tachyarrhythmias or "silent atria." Usually, VVI pacing is selected for patients with AV block and chronic or paroxysmal atrial tachyarrhythmias. The addition of rate modulation (AAIR or VVIR) is indicated when sinus node function is abnormal. Chronotropic incompetence is a common form of abnormal sinus node function in which appropriate increases in sinus rate do not occur.

The AAT modality is rarely used but does have application in the assessment of atrial sensing with some DDD devices in patients who are not pacemaker dependent. For example, after reprogramming to the AAT mode with an atrial rate less than sinus rate and a relatively low unipolar atrial output (≤1.0 V), the atrial sensitivity setting is progressively reprogrammed from the least to the most sensitive values while simultaneously observing the ECG. As soon as atrial sensing is reached, "triggered" atrial stimuli will begin to appear within the P wave on the ECG. Until then (at less sensitive values), one will observe atrial stimuli at the programmed rate that are dissociated from the native P waves. In this way, one can determine at what level atrial sensing occurs and program the appropriate sensitivity. In some of the more recent pacemakers, built-in automatic sensing threshold determination is a standard feature. Similarly, the VVT mode is rarely used except when trying to elicit diagnostic information, such as any extraneous electric activity that may be sensed by the pacemaker through the ventricular lead. Again, this would be performed in patients with DDD devices who are not pacemaker dependent and only after turning the ventricular output down to a lower level.

DUAL-CHAMBER PERMANENT PACEMAKERS

Pacemaker Timing Cycles (Intervals)

A given pacemaker's sensing and pacing behavior can be expressed in terms of *timing cycles*. The simplest way to appreciate timing cycles is to examine the behavior of a DDD pacemaker at its lower rate limit. This situation occurs when both spontaneous atrial and ventricular activity are slower than the programmed lower rate limit of the pacemaker (Fig. 5-1). The intervals usually are expressed in milliseconds.

The *basic interval* is the time between two consecutive paced events without an intervening sensed event. It is also known as the *automatic, demand,* or *pac-*

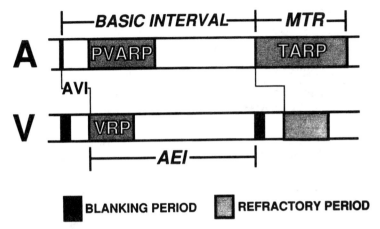

FIG. 5-1. Basic timing cycles for both the atrial chamber (upper panel) and the ventricular chamber (lower panel). Note that the lower rate limit is the sum of the AV interval (*AVI*) and the atrial escape interval (*AEI*). The upper rate limit is equivalent to the total atrial refractory period (*TARP*), which is the sum of the AVI and the PVARP. (VRP = ventricular refractory period; *MTR*, maximum tracking rate.) See text for explanation.

ing interval. In Figure 5-1, the basic interval is shown for a DDD device functioning at its lower rate limit (LRL).

The *blanking period* is a brief interval initiated by an output pulse during which sensing cannot occur. Typically, an atrial stimulus disables ventricular sensing for a 25- to 35-msec period to prevent inadvertent sensing of the atrial stimulus by the ventricular channel, thereby preventing inappropriate inhibition of ventricular output. Were this not to occur, "cross-talk" between the atrial and ventricular channels might lead to absent ventricular stimulation.

The *AV interval* (AVI) is the interval between either an atrial sensed or an atrial paced event and the delivery of a ventricular stimulus. The interval is usually programmed to 150 to 220 msec but may be lengthened to allow for native AV conduction in cases of long PR intervals. During the AVI, the atrial channel is refractory to any sensed events and thus constitutes a portion of the atrial refractory period.

The *postventricular atrial refractory period* (PVARP) is a period of atrial refractoriness that extends beyond the delivery of a ventricular stimulus or beyond a ventricular sensed event. In a way, it is the atrial equivalent of the ventricular blanking period, in which the disabling of sensing is taking place in the atrial channel. Its primary purpose is to prevent pacemaker-mediated tachycardia by ignoring retrogradely conducted atrial impulses.

The *total atrial refractory period* (TARP) is the sum of the AVI and the PVARP. During this period, atrial events cannot be sensed. The TARP also determines the pacemaker's upper rate limit.

The *atrial escape interval* (AEI) is the interval that begins with a ventricular sensed or paced event and ends with an atrial paced event. The LRL of the DDD pacemaker equals the AVI plus the AEI. The AEI is also known as the *VA interval*. In a DDD device, any sensed atrial event occurring after the PVARP but before the AEI is completed will be sensed and followed by the AVI unless a spontaneously conducted QRS occurs first. As discussed later, the DVI pacemaker will not respond to such a P wave by prematurely ending the AEI. Because atrial sensing is absent, the AEI is allowed to be completed and ends with the next expected atrial stimulus. Because atrial sensing does not occur, the opportunity exists for competition between native and paced atrial activity; on occasion, this can be arrhythmogenic. In the case of a DDI pacemaker, the atrial event is sensed, but because of the inhibitory function, the next atrial output pulse is suppressed. As in the DVI mode, the AEI is allowed to complete, after which the AV interval is begun. Unless a spontaneously conducted QRS complex occurs before the end of the AVI, a ventricular stimulus then is delivered at the time determined by the LRL. The VDD device operates identically to the DDD pacemaker. Thus, the DVI, DDI, and VDD (or DDD) can be distinguished from each other on the basis of their response to a sensed atrial event during the AEI.

The *ventricular refractory period* (VRP) is an interval initiated by the ventricular sensed or paced event during which there is no ventricular sensing. It differs from the ventricular blanking period in that it is initiated by a ventricular sensed event, not an atrial sensed event as in the blanking period.

The *upper rate limit* of dual-chamber pacemakers represents the highest ventricular pacing rate that can be achieved in response to atrial sensed events and still maintain 1 to 1 AV synchrony at the programmed AV delay. This is also known as the *maximum tracking rate* (MTR). The limit of the MTR is the TARP. In other words, a 1 to 1 AV response will not occur if the upper rate limit interval is programmed to be shorter than the TARP. Most DDD programmers will automatically calculate the MTR based on the selections of the AVI and the PVARP. If the inadvertently selected MTR is shorter than the TARP, the device usually will signal this fact so that the appropriate changes can be made. The manner in which the AV response changes once the MTR is exceeded depends on the device. Either a 2 to 1 AV response will occur, or a Wenckebach pattern results. Rate smoothing is a variation of upper rate behavior that prevents marked changes in cycle length anytime the MTR is exceeded, whether produced by a single premature atrial beat or by a gradually increasing sinus rate. Because rate smoothing is a response of the ventricular output only, "smoothing" of the ventricular rate is achieved sometimes at the expense of losing AV synchrony. The benefit of this feature is a decrease in the subjective sensation of abrupt changes in heart rate that the patient may experience.

Commonly Used Dual-chamber Modes

VDD

The VDD mode provides for what is commonly known as P wave or atrial synchronous pacing. As long as there is a stable sinus rhythm with a rate above the LRL of the device, each P wave is sensed and is followed by the programmed AV interval, ending with a delivered ventricular stimulus. Figure 5-2A shows an example of the response to a premature atrial beat occurring within the AEI. In this example, the premature P wave occurs beyond PVARP, and so it is sensed and followed by the programmed AV interval. The second tracing shows the response to a premature ventricular beat within intact retrograde conduction. The

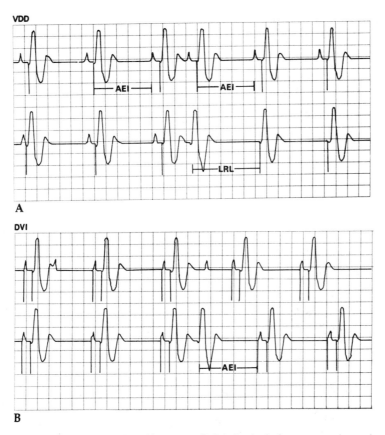

FIG. 5-2. Representative examples of lower rate limit behavior in four commonly used modes: VDD (**A**), DVI (**B**), DDI (**C**), DDD (**D**). In each example, the upper tracing represents the response of the pacemaker to a premature atrial beat; the lower tracing represents the response to a premature ventricular beat. See text for explanation.

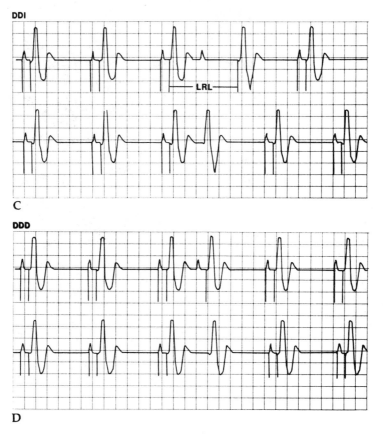

FIG. 5-2. *Continued.*

retrograde P wave occurs within PVARP and therefore is not sensed. Because the timing of the next sinus P wave exceeds the LRL, the next event is a ventricular paced beat. P-wave tracking will resume as soon as the next P wave occurs outside PVARP.

DVI

Also known as *AV sequential pacing*, DVI provides for pacing in both atrium and ventricle but sensing only in the ventricle. The inhibitory function always serves to inhibit the ventricular output. If an R wave is sensed during the atrial escape interval, the atrial output is also inhibited. Figure 5-2B illustrates the effect of a premature atrial (upper tracing) and a premature ventricular beat (lower tracing). In the upper tracing, AV pacing is undisturbed by the presence of the premature atrial beat. In the lower tracing, the premature ventricular beat is sensed and inhibits both the atrial and ventricular outputs. The AEI is reset, and the next atrial paced beat occurs at the end of the new AEI.

Two points are worth mentioning with regard to the DVI mode. One is that competition between native P waves and paced P waves can occur and may result in the induction of atrial arrhythmias. The second is that the DVI mode is useful in preventing pacemaker-mediated tachycardia. This problem occurs when a ventricular paced beat results in retrograde AV nodal conduction and produces a premature P wave. If this premature P wave were sensed, a ventricular output would follow the usual AV interval, and a vicious cycle would be established, resulting in pacemaker-induced tachycardia. Reprogramming a DDD pacemaker to the DVI mode is one way to prevent this problem, but the usual approach is to lengthen the programmable feature, PVARP.

DDI

Usually referred to as *AV sequential, non-P-synchronous pacing with dual-chamber sensing*, DDI is similar to DVI pacing except that it incorporates atrial sensing in addition to ventricular sensing and therefore prevents competitive atrial pacing. In this mode, any atrial event following PVARP is sensed, but no atrial pacing is delivered at the end of the AEI, thus eliminating atrial competition. The timing of the next ventricular stimulus is determined by the LRL of the pacemaker. Examples of a response to a premature atrial (upper tracing) and ventricular (lower tracing) beat are shown in Figure 5-2C. In the upper tracing, the premature atrial beat occurs after PVARP and is sensed, but no atrial paced output is delivered at the end of the AEI (as would occur in the DVI mode). Instead, a ventricular output is delivered on reaching the established LRL. In the lower tracing, the premature ventricular beat is sensed and inhibits further ventricular output until the LRL is reached. The advantage of the DDI mode is in situations where paroxysmal atrial tachyarrhythmias occur. Because sensed atrial activity occurring faster than the LRL has an inhibitory function, the pacemaker begins ventricular pacing at the LRL.

DDD

Known as the *fully automatic pacemaker*, DDD is capable of sensing and pacing in both the atrium and ventricle. It is the dual-chamber device with the fewest drawbacks. The upper tracing in Figure 5-2D shows the response of a DDD device to a premature atrial beat occurring within the AEI. The sensed atrial event is followed by a ventricular paced output after the programmed AVI. This behavior is identical to that of the VDD mode. In the lower tracing, the premature ventricular beat is sensed and, in the absence of any VA conduction, the next atrial paced stimulus occurs on completion of the AEI. This is followed by the delivery of a ventricular stimulus determined by the programmed AV interval.

Upper rate behavior differs according to the mode. In the VDD mode, when the sensed atrial rate exceeds the upper rate limit, either 2-to-1 or Wenckebach AV conduction begins with a ventricular response dependent on the atrial rate. The DDD mode operates in the same fashion. For both DVI and DDI, upper rate limit behavior is not really applicable, either because atrial activity is not sensed (DVI) or because any sensed atrial activity results in inhibition of atrial output (DDI). When there is a sudden increase in atrial rate, the DVI device will continue to pace both atrium and ventricle at the LRL. In the DDI mode, only ventricular pacing at the LRL occurs. Thus, only when the letter *D* occupies the third position in the code will there be an ability to program for upper rate limit behavior. A summary of the sensing operation, indications, and relative contraindications of the various pacemakers is provided in Figure 5-3.

Benefits of Maintaining Atrioventricular Synchrony

Attempts to mimic normal atrial and ventricular electric activation of the heart with artificial pacemakers are more than two decades old, and yet permanent AV cardiac pacing has become reliable only with recent advances in pulse-generator technology, battery longevity, and atrial lead systems. The benefits of maintaining AV synchrony through use of an atrial pacemaker or a dual-chamber pacemaker are discussed in the following sections.

Physiologic Timing of Atrioventricular Valve Closure

With the VVI, the possibility exists of poorly timed atrial contraction in relation to ventricular contraction. If the atria contract at the same time that the ventricles contract, mitral and tricuspid valve regurgitation may result, with subsequent low cardiac output and pulmonary congestion. Another manifestation associated with absent AV synchrony is the *pacemaker syndrome*, which is caused by single-chamber ventricular pacing and may have a variety of symptoms including malaise, easy fatigability, light-headedness, and, less commonly, syncope. Most of these symptoms are due to the lower blood pressure and cardiac output that often exist during VVI pacing. Symptoms resulting from elevated atrial and venous pressures may include dyspnea–orthopnea, neck fullness, early satiety, and, occasionally, peripheral edema. Pacemaker syndrome can be related to simple AV dissociation or to the periodic development of retrograde AV nodal conduction. One must always remember that the symptoms that were supposed to be alleviated by the implant may recur in the form of pacemaker syndrome. Also, any new symptoms suggesting impaired cardiac performance following pacemaker insertion should raise the possibility of this syndrome, which usually is alleviated by an upgrade to a DDD device. Improved timing of AV conduction also may be useful in patients with marked PR interval prolongation.

PACEMAKER TYPE	INDICATIONS	LIMITATIONS / CONTRAINDICATIONS
A VVI Ventricular Demand	Significant Bradycardia With: 1. Normal Sinus Rhythm with only rare episodes of A-V block or sinus arrest. 2. Chronic atrial fibrillation. 3. Severe physical disability. 4. Concurrence of another disease with short prognosis.	1. Patients who do not have specified indications for VVI and who may benefit from physiological pacing. 2. Hemodynamic compromise due to VVI induced retrograde A-V conduction.
B AAI Atrial Demand	1. SSS with symptoms. 2. Control of bradycardia due to drug therapy.	1. Overt AVB. 2. Occult AVB. a. HV > 55 ms; b. HV prolongation with increasing atrial drive rate to 180 ppm; c. 2° Mobitz 1 AVB at < 140 ppm atrial drive rate ; d. Bifascicular block. 3. Chronic atrial flutter/fibrillation. 4. Atrial fibrillation or inability to stimulate the atrium.
C VAT P-Wave Synchronous	1. AVB without SSS.	1. Atrial fibrillation, flutter. 2. SSS. 3. Slow retrograde A-V conduction. 4. Sinus rhythm with rare episodes of AVB. 5. Pacemaker can be competitive with ventricular extrasystoles. 6. Pacemaker fails to maintain synchrony below lower tracking rate.
D VDD P-Wave Synchronous	1. AVB without SSS.	1. Atrial fibrillation, flutter — intermittent or chronic. 2. SSS. 3. Slow retrograde A-V conduction. 4. Sinus rhythm with rare episodes of AVB. 5. Pacemaker fails to maintain synchrony below lower tracking rate.
E DVI A-V Sequential	1. AVB with additional findings of SSS. 2. SSS with additional findings of AVB.	1. Chronic atrial fibrillation, flutter. 2. Lacks physiological rate responsiveness. 3. Competitive atrial stimulation.
F DDD Fully Automatic	1. Atrial Bradyarrhythmias with or without AVB. 2. Normal sinus rhythm with AVB.	1. Chronic atrial fibrillation, flutter. 2. Paroxysmal atrial tachyarrhythmias. 3. Slow retrograde A-V conduction.

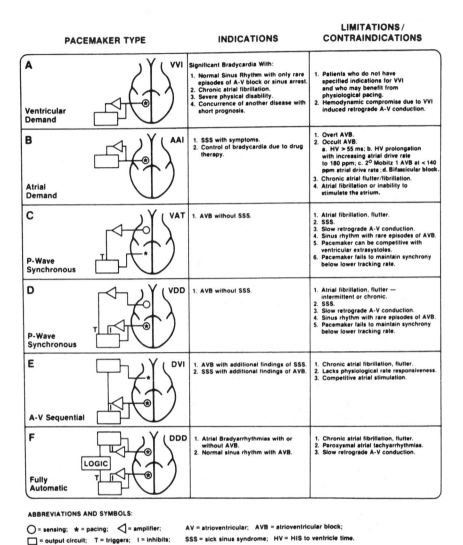

ABBREVIATIONS AND SYMBOLS:

○ = sensing; ★ = pacing; ◁ = amplifier; AV = atrioventricular; AVB = atrioventricular block;

□ = output circuit; T = triggers; I = inhibits; SSS = sick sinus syndrome; HV = HIS to ventricle time.

FIG. 5-3. Diagrammatic representation of pacing modes. The left-hand column illustrates attachment of the amplifier and output circuit to the right ventricle or right atrium by the pacing lead. The major indications and the major limitations and contraindications for the types of pacing demonstrated are listed. (Courtesy of Drs. Richard Sutton and Paul Citron.)

Improved Cardiac Output

An increase in stroke volume and cardiac output occurs when ventricular filling is augmented by atrial contraction as a result of the Frank–Starling relationship. When the atrium contracts, ventricular volume at the end of diastole is greater so that the ventricle begins its contraction higher on its function curve (Fig. 5-4). Augmentation of ventricular stroke volume by atrial contraction is most important in stiff, noncompliant hearts, as may be seen in patients with congestive heart failure, aortic stenosis, or hypertension. The improved stroke volume with properly timed atrial contraction carries no significant additional myocardial oxygen demand and, in addition, allows the heart to work higher on its ventricular function curve without an appreciable increase in mean pulmonary capillary pressure. Thus, the improved cardiac output occurs without increased risk for pulmonary congestion.

Possible Decrease in Tachycardias

Maintaining AV synchrony with use of an atrial or a dual-chamber pacemaker may reduce tachycardias in selected patients. This benefit is not as well established as are avoidance of simultaneous atrial and ventricular contraction and increased cardiac output.

The clinician is faced with complex decisions regarding the type of pacemaker to place. An algorithm adapted from one originally designed by Paul Levine, M.D., is provided in Figure 5-5.

Additional considerations may need to be made in arriving at a final decision. Patients who require infrequent pacing should be considered for implantation of a VVI device that exhibits hysteresis. That is, the LRL may be 50 bpm, but the patient is allowed to decrease to 40 bpm before the device begins pacing (at a rate of 50 bpm). Patients in whom there is evidence of diastolic dysfunction (e.g., in patients who have had a prior myocardial infarction, chronic hypertensive heart disease, hypertrophic cardiomyopathy, or echocardiographic evidence of a stiff left ventricle) always should be considered candidates for dual-chamber pacing. In any patient with chronotropic incompetence, an effort should be made to main-

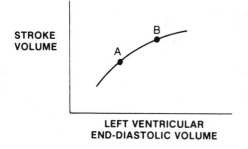

STROKE VOLUME

LEFT VENTRICULAR END-DIASTOLIC VOLUME

FIG. 5-4. Frank–Starling curve. In this example, at point A the patient does not have an atrial kick, the left ventricular end-diastolic volume is relatively small, and the stroke volume poor. At point B, the atrial kick has returned, the end-diastolic volume is increased, and the stroke volume is increased. This occurs with no significant increase in oxygen consumption.

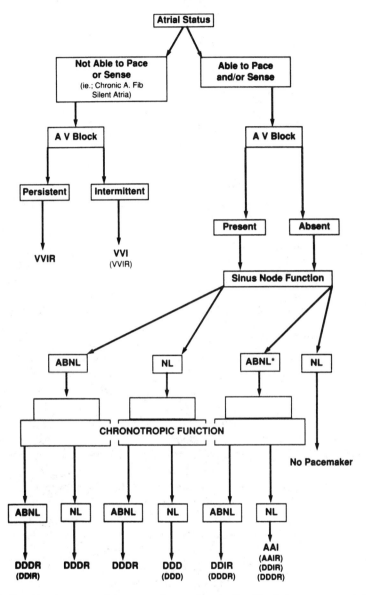

FIG. 5-5. Algorithm for appropriate pacemaker mode selection (*Includes paroxysmal atrial fibrillation or flutter).

tain AV synchrony as well as incorporate the rate-modulated feature. Whereas it is not always possible to determine before pacemaker implantation, any evidence for a predisposition to pacemaker syndrome should be treated by selecting a dual-chamber device. Patients who remain quite active should be strongly considered for rate modulation. Finally, in significantly debilitated patients, those with short life expectancy (less than 1 year), or patients in whom mental competence is questioned, a single-chamber device may be more sensible than a dual-chamber one. The additional cost associated with a dual-chamber device may provide no additional improvements in the quality of the patient's life.

TEMPORARY PACEMAKER APPLICATION

Transvenous Temporary Pacing

The most commonly used temporary pacemaker is the single-chamber pacemaker that is usually used for ventricular pacing (VVI). A no. 6 French bipolar or quadripolar electrode catheter is most commonly used. The catheter tip is advanced into the right ventricular apex under fluoroscopic guidance and secured to minimize tip migration. In contrast to the traditional anteroposterior (AP) projection, the right anterior oblique (RAO) is a much safer approach in that the tip movement toward the right ventricular apex can be better appreciated. By advancing the catheter tip in the AP projection, one may not know that the tip is not responding to the advancing motions, and the risk of perforation is thus greater. The temporary device is set with three variables in mind: rate, pulse output, and sensitivity. If AV block is intermittent, it is usually best to set the rate to a value below the spontaneous ventricular rate to preserve normal AV synchrony. In some situations, however, it may be desirable to pace the heart at a faster rate (80–100 bpm) to assist in the maintenance of an adequate blood pressure. The capture threshold always should be determined at the time of catheter placement because this value can be compared with later determinations in the event of suspected dislodgement. Capture threshold is determined by pacing at a rate faster than the spontaneous ventricular rate and gradually turning the output down from 4 to 5 mA to the value at which noncapture occurs. This value is noted as a threshold, and the output is turned back up to at least twice this value. The sensitivity setting is usually left in the "demand" setting, which is a fully clockwise rotation of the dial. The electrode catheter should be secured firmly near its exit from the intravascular sheath through which it was placed. Common routes of placement include the femoral, subclavian, or internal jugular approaches. Maintenance of sterility can be a problem when using the femoral approach compared with using the other sites.

Single-chamber atrial pacing using a J-lead is appropriate only in situations of sinus bradycardia in the absence of the AV block. Dual-chamber temporary pacing is becoming increasingly common. The additional variable to set at the time of placement is the AV interval. Values of 150 to 200 msec are common. It is important to remember that in any patient in whom permanent pacemaker implantation is contemplated, the subclavian routes should be avoided if at all possible.

Transcutaneous Temporary Pacing

The traditional approach of transvenous pacing generally requires fluoroscopy and, often, transport of the patient to a fluoroscopy suite, with significant delay. The transthoracic approach of placing a needle directly into the heart on an emergency basis carries considerable risk and is often ineffective. Therefore, transcutaneous pacing has recently made a "comeback." This approach, originally developed by Dr. P. M. Zoll, did not become widely popular initially because of considerable pain associated with the transcutaneous pacemaker. The development of large pads that disburse the electric current over a wide surface area and the use of a wide pulse width have reduced the pain of cutaneous nerve and skeletal muscle stimulation and revived interest in this approach (Fig. 5-6). As with other forms of resuscitation, this is not a particularly effective mode of therapy in a patient who has undergone cardiopulmonary resuscitation for a prolonged period and whose asystole is the result of advanced myocardial damage.

The typical transcutaneous pacing device generates a current that can be increased from approximately 40 mA up to 200 mA. The average-size adult usu-

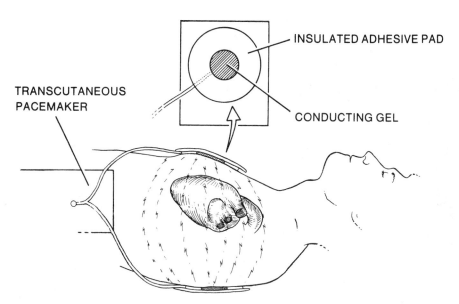

FIG. 5-6. Transcutaneous temporary pacing. Current is passed through the thorax of a patient attached to a transcutaneous pacemaker.

ally can be paced with a current of 40 to 70 mA. (A transvenous pacemaker will usually capture the heart at less than 1 or 2 mA.) The higher levels of current are painful, even with the broad pads disbursing the charge. The pulse width is approximately 20 to 30 msec long, compared with a permanent pacemaker with a pulse width of 0.5 msec. Generally, the pads are placed on the front and back of the chest so that the current travels across the myocardium to stimulate it (Fig. 5-7). Several devices with varying abilities to sense the patient's intrinsic heart rhythm are available commercially. Often these are kept on a cart with a defibrillator because they may be used in the setting of cardiac arrest.

The transcutaneous pacemaker generates much current, which creates problems with performing electrocardiography or monitoring. The monitor strip on the device itself does not measure the actual pacemaker spike but rather causes a deflection on the ECG paper during the pacemaker spike, thus avoiding excessive deflection of the ECG stylus. This can create a misleading situation. Even if the pads are not attached to the patient, deflection will occur, giving the appearance that a spike is being generated on the patient. It is often difficult to judge

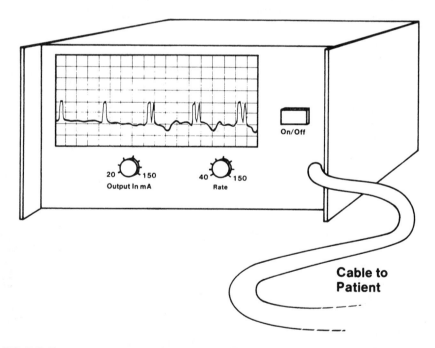

FIG. 5-7. Transcutaneous pacemaker generator. The transcutaneous pacemaker generator is attached to a cable with two pads that are attached to the patient to complete the circuit, with current transmitted across the patient's thorax. In this hypothetical generator, the output can be adjusted to the minimum amount of current required to effect capture, thereby reducing patient discomfort. The pacing rate can be adjusted also. Attachments could be available for esophageal pacing.

from the ECG or rhythm strip whether the heart is actually being captured. The patient's pulse can be palpated during the use of the transcutaneous pacemaker, which does not result in any shock if the femoral or carotid pulse is well away from the current between the two electrodes. Putting the hand between the electrodes can result in a shock. Palpating the pulse is an effective way of determining whether capture is occurring.

When the patient is being monitored on a standard ECG monitoring system in an intensive care unit, the gain is generally turned to the lowest possible level because of the large pacemaker spike. This can create confusion when the pacemaker is turned off to assess underlying rhythm. The patient's baseline may appear to be a straight line or have minor changes resembling P waves that may be QRS complexes. Palpating the patient's pulse can help clarify this, as can turning up the gain on the monitor for a more visible QRS signal (Fig. 5-8).

Potential problems with transthoracic pacing include poor capture if the patient is extremely large or has significant transthoracic resistance to electric stimulation. Ventricular capture may not be possible from external patches at a

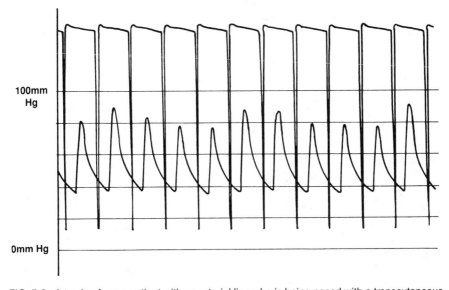

FIG. 5-8. A tracing from a patient with an arterial line who is being paced with a transcutaneous pacemaker. The patient had presented with dramatic, severe asystole and responded to transcutaneous pacemaking emergently. The patient's blood pressure is about 85/40 and is stabilized with the transcutaneous pacemaker. Note the size of the transcutaneous pacemaker spikes, which were greater than 11 cm in height with routine standardization. The QRS complex is not easily noted, but 1-to-1 pacing is documented with the arterial line. If the massive transcutaneous pacing spike were shrunk down for a routine bedside monitor, the QRS complex would be essentially invisible and monitoring would be difficult. The value of arterial monitoring is obvious. We encountered a situation in which the transcutaneous pacemaker was believed not to be working because of the virtually invisible QRS complex after the massive spike.

pacing amplitude that is comfortable to the patient. At the same time, some patients do not tolerate even the minimal requirements for pacing thresholds and have requested removal of this type of pacing device.

Other considerations for an external pacing device include those situations in which a transvenous pacemaker is absolutely or relatively contraindicated such as (a) hemorrhagic status, (b) tricuspid valve prosthesis, (c) existing endocarditis or infected endocardial pacemaker lead, (d) sepsis or bacteremia, (e) bone marrow suppression, (f) immune deficiency, and (g) ventricular tachycardia associated with digitalis toxicity. Our practice has been to place a transvenous pacemaker fairly soon after the transcutaneous pacemaker has stabilized the patient because of lack of experience with prolonged transcutaneous pacing.

A transcutaneous pacemaker always should be in place when AV junctional ablation is being carried out to create complete AV block. This provides a suitable backup if the temporary transvenous system malfunctions initially.

Esophageal Pacing

A method for pacing the atria on a temporary basis using a less invasive technique than that of a transvenous pacemaker has been developed through the use of esophageal pacing electrodes. The proximity of the atria to the esophagus has been used in the past for atrial electrogram recordings to help determine what type of cardiac rhythm a patient may be in, be it atrial flutter, atrial fibrillation, or some type of AV or AV nodal reentrant tachycardia. Typically, the pulse amplitude used in esophageal pacing is on the order of 15 to 20 mA and the pulse width is 10-20 msec.

Transesophageal pacing is usually more effective in pacing the atrium than the ventricle because the former structure is closer to the esophagus. The lowest effective pulse amplitude is chosen to minimize any potential discomfort.

The following are indications for transesophageal recording and pacing: (a) for the assessment of normal atrial or sinus rhythm recording versus atrial fibrillation or atrial flutter during time periods of unknown cardiac rhythm; (b) to determine whether a patient has any potential for ventricular preexcitation [Wolff–Parkinson–White (WPW) versus Mahaim fiber]; (c) for the assessment of sinus node activity through the performance of sinus node recovery times; (d) for overdrive pacing of atrial flutter to sinus rhythm; (e) as backup pacing for patients with bradycardia with an intact AV conduction system; (f) as potential for overdrive pacing of the atria to help suppress ventricular arrhythmias; and (g) for potential for induction of supraventricular arrhythmias and assessment of AV conduction.

A standard bipolar transvenous catheter with an interelectrode distance of 15 to 30 mm is most often used. This can be a standard electrode distance as seen in a bipolar pacemaker, or quadripolar pacemakers may be used using combinations of electrodes 2 cm or more apart. Often the use of electrode distances of 2 cm apart may not be optimal, and the use of electrode combinations of 3 cm or more apart may be necessary. The amount of current necessary using a 10-msec pulse duration is usually 10 to 15 mA.

Placement of the esophageal recording/pacing electrode catheter is similar to that of the nasogastric tube but is usually less difficult because of its smaller diameter. The patient should be seated in an upright position to minimize apprehension. The catheter tip is lubricated with 2% lidocaine (Xylocaine) jelly to minimize nasopharyngeal discomfort. The posterior oral pharynx should be lightly sprayed with an aerosolized local anesthetic. The catheter tip should be advanced through the nare so that it follows along the floor of the nasal passages. After turning inferiorly on reaching the posterior nasopharynx, the catheter tip usually will elicit a mild gagging sensation. At this point, the patient should be instructed to take several small sips from a glass of water through a straw while simultaneously, and quickly, the catheter is advanced. Paroxysms of cough usually indicate that the catheter tip may have inadvertently entered the trachea and should be withdrawn. The tip should be advanced to approximately 35 to 40 cm from the nare and recordings taken. At least two channels should be displayed, one for the esophageal electrogram and the other a surface lead. The purpose of the surface lead is to establish the timing of ventricular activation. The catheter then is withdrawn slowly and the esophageal electrogram tracing observed for the appearance of atrial deflections. The timing of the atrial deflections will differ from that of the QRS complex observed on the surface lead.

When the pacing begins, it must be noted that not only can atrial pacing commence but also ventricular pacing can occur, and the clinician must be aware that ventricular arrhythmias can develop. Therefore, it is recommended that a defibrillator be available on standby. During pacing, the patient frequently will describe a sensation of gastroesophageal reflux or complain of indigestion.

REFERENCES

Baig MW, Perrins EJ. The hemodynamics of cardiac pacing: clinical and physiological aspects. *Prog Cardiovasc Dis* 1991;33:283.

Barold SS. The DDI mode of cardiac pacing (Part I). *Pacing Clin Electrophysiol* 1987;10:480.

Barold SS. Transesophageal pacing. *Pacing Clin Electrophysiol* 1990;13:1324.

Bedotto JB, Grayburn PA, Black WH, et al. Alterations in left ventricular relaxation during atrioventricular pacing in humans. *J Am Coll Cardiol* 1990;15:658.

Dreifus LS. Choosing the optimal cardiac pacemaker. *Am Coll Cardiol Highlights* 1985;1:1.

Eugene M, Lascault G, Frank R, et al. Assessment of the optimal atrioventricular delay in DDD paced patients by impedance plethysmography. *Eur Heart J* 1989;10:250.

Jahangir A, Shen W, Neubauer S, et al. Relation between mode of pacing and long-term survival in the very elderly. *J Am Coll Cardiol* 1999;33:1208.

Liebert HP, O'Donoghue S, Tullner WF, Platia EV. Pacemaker syndrome in activity-responsive VVI pacing. *Am J Cardiol* 1989;64:124.

Mabo P, Pouillot C, Kermarrec A, et al. Lack of physiological adaptation of the atrioventricular interval to heart rate in patients chronically paced in the AAIR mode. *Pacing Clin Electrophysiol* 1991;14:2133.

Madsen JK, Meibom J, Videbak R, et al. Transcutaneous pacing: experience with the Zoll noninvasive temporary pacemaker. *Am Heart J* 1988;116:7.

Ritter P, Daubert C, Mabo P, et al. Hemodynamic benefit of a rate-adapted A-V delay in dual chamber pacing. *Eur Heart J* 1989;10:637.

Rokey R, Quinones MA, Zoghbi WA, et al. Influence of left atrial systolic emptying on left ventricular early filling dynamics by Doppler in patients with sequential atrioventricular pacemakers. *Am J Cardiol* 1988;62:968.

Rosenqvist M, Obel IWP. Atrial pacing and the risk for AV block: is there a time for change in attitude (Part I)? *Pacing Clin Electrophysiol* 1989;12:97.

Ryden L. Atrial inhibited pacing—An underused mode of cardiac stimulation. *Pacing Clin Electrophysiol* 1988;11:1375.

Ryden L, Karlsson O, Kristensson B-E. The importance of different atrioventricular intervals for exercise capacity. *Pacing Clin Electrophysiol* 1988;11:1051.

Santini M, Ansalone G, Cacciatore G, Turitto G. Transesophageal pacing. *Pacing Clin Electrophysiol* 1990;13:1298.

Zoll PM. Noninvasive cardiac stimulation revisited (Part II). *Pacing Clin Electrophysiol* 1990;13:2014.

6

Dual-chamber Pacing: Special Considerations

With the information discussed in Chapter 5, we now can take a closer look at some of the features unique to dual-chamber pacing.

CROSS-TALK AND VENTRICULAR SAFETY PACING

In a dual-chamber pacing system with atrial and ventricular pacing and ventricular sensing, the atrial pacemaker spike or its after-potential could be sensed by the ventricular system and inhibit ventricular firing (the ventricular system might interpret the atrial event as a ventricular contraction). This occurrence is referred to as *cross-talk*, and pacemakers are designed to avoid cross-talk using various methods. Cross-talk is more likely to occur if the atrial lead is unipolar (because of the large spike and after-potential) than if it is bipolar.

One approach to preventing cross-talk is using the committed pacemaker, a type of dual-chamber pacemaker in which the ventricular system is committed to fire once the atrial system fires. Even if a premature ventricular contraction (PVC) occurs after the atrial lead has fired, the PVC will not be sensed and the ventricular system will fire into the PVC. This design is particularly useful in a dual-chamber system with unipolar leads (but unipolar DDD pacing is rarely, if ever, used now). A theoretic disadvantage is that the ventricular spike could be placed just after a PVC; however, this has not been shown to be a practical problem because the atrioventricular (AV) spike-to-spike interval is so short (usually approximately 150 msec) that the ventricular pacemaker spike does not fall on the T wave of the PVC, and pacemaker-induced ventricular tachycardia has not been a problem.

Another approach to cross-talk is so-called ventricular safety pacing. In such pacing, if the ventricular lead senses an event that it would interpret as ventricular depolarization, the ventricular lead fires somewhat earlier than the preset AV delay. If the ventricular lead senses the atrial spike firing, this still results in ventricular depolarization. If it senses a PVC occurring after the atrial lead has

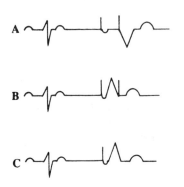

FIG. 6-1. Committed and noncommitted dual-chamber pacing. **A:** Intrinsic sinus beat followed by atrial and ventricular sequential pacing. This could be either a committed or a noncommitted pacemaker. **B:** Intrinsic sinus beat followed by atrial pacing with capture of the atrium. A premature ventricular contraction (*PVC*) occurs just after the P wave. This is a committed system, and the pacemaker spike falls at the end of the PVC. This represents normal function of a committed pacemaker system. The spike-to-spike interval is relatively short, and the pacemaker spike does not fall on the T wave of the PVC. **C:** Intrinsic sinus beat followed by a paced atrial beat and a PVC. This is a noncommitted system. The PVC is sensed and the ventricular system is inhibited. This is normal functioning of a noncommitted dual-chamber pacing system.

fired, it simply causes a spike to appear toward the end of the QRS complex of the PVC and thus decreases the likelihood that a spike would appear on the Q wave of the PVC. This may add a degree of safety to a DDD pacemaker; however, it increases the complexity of interpretation of the pacemaker electrocardiogram (ECG).

A noncommitted pacemaker is a dual-chamber pacemaker in which the ventricular system can sense a ventricular contraction and be inhibited even after the atrial system has fired. In this type of pacemaker, cross-talk can be avoided by use of a blanking period. For several milliseconds during and after the firing of the atrial system, the ventricular system is not inhibited by the electric activity— the blanking period—thus avoiding inappropriate inhibition of the ventricular system by the atrial system (Fig. 6-1).

PACEMAKER-MEDIATED TACHYCARDIA

Figure 6-2 demonstrates a pacemaker-mediated arrhythmia that has been referred to as an *endless loop*. In either a VDD or DDD pacemaker, sensing occurs in the atrium and triggers the ventricle. Retrograde AV [ventricle-to-atrium (V-A)] conduction occurs in response to ventricular pacing, which causes atrial contraction, shown schematically as an inverted P wave in Figure 6-2. (Do not expect the P wave to be so readily visible in clinical practice.) Sensing of the P wave causes the ventricle to be stimulated, completing the endless loop or circus tachycardia.

Figure 6-2 shows the problem of slow retrograde AV conduction. If the V-A conduction occurred rapidly, it would tend to fall into the atrial refractory period, during which atrial sensing does not occur, and no endless loop arrhythmias would occur. The length of the atrial refractory period varies from model to model and always should be programmable in modern DDD pacemakers. It extends from the atrial spike to beyond the QRS complex.

Not all patients have V-A conduction, but some patients with complete antegrade AV block may have intact retrograde AV conduction. Electrophysiologic

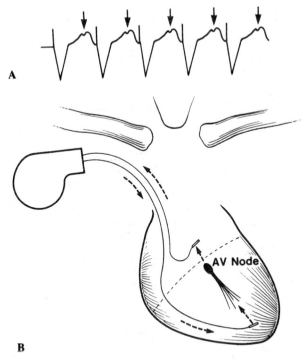

FIG. 6-2. Endless loop or circus tachycardia. **A:** In this dual-chamber pacemaker, sensing occurs in the atrium that triggers a ventricular spike after an appropriate delay. The ventricular rate is at or near the upper rate limit of the DDD pacemaker. Ventricular depolarization is followed by a retrograde P wave as a result of ventricular–atrial conduction (demonstrated as an exaggerated inverted P wave marked by an arrow). The retrograde P wave sensed in the atrium causes the ventricle to fire again, and this creates a pacemaker-mediated tachycardia. It is generally treated by eliminating sensing the retrograde P wave. This is a DDD pacemaker that is firing at or near the upper rate limit in the ventricle (due to the sensed retrograde P waves). **B:** Diagrammatic representation of the mechanism of endless loop tachycardia.

testing for V-A conduction before implantation of a DDD or VDD unit is useful, but the V-A conduction may be intermittent.

Two approaches can be used to stop the pacemaker-mediated tachycardia (PMT):

1. Block V-A conduction (usually not successful).
    a. Natural fatigue of the retrograde pathway may occur, causing spontaneous termination.
    b. Carotid sinus massage may block V-A conduction.
    c. The use of drugs such as digoxin or verapamil is almost never successful and may in fact cause PMT by slowing V-A conduction, thus allowing sensing of a retrograde P wave occurring after the atrial refractory period.
2. Block sensing in the atrium.
    a. Applying a magnet stops atrial sensing and interrupts PMT

   b. Extending the atrial refractory period is the most commonly successful method of stopping PMT.

   c. Reprogramming the DDD or VDD pacemaker to VVI or DVI stops atrial sensing and eliminates the possibility of PMT. Programming to DDI eliminates the triggered response in the ventricle. This can be coupled with DDI-R to maintain rate responsiveness.

   d. One manufacturer programs the pacemaker not to sense the sixteenth beat if the unit is running at or near its upper rate limit, thus interrupting PMT but not causing problems if the rapid rate is caused by sinus tachycardia.

   e. The pacemaker can be designed to extend automatically the atrial refractory period after a PVC, thereby reducing the likelihood that PMT will develop since it may begin due to retrograde atrioventricular conduction after a PVC.

UPPER RATE LIMIT

Pacemakers in which the ventricle is stimulated in response to atrial sensing present a special problem with high atrial rates. Such pacemakers need a method of handling high atrial rates so that the presence of episodes such as atrial flutter or atrial tachycardia do not result in a dangerously rapid ventricular response.

One approach to upper rate limit is for the pacemaker abruptly to develop 2:1 block at the upper rate limit. If a patient developed atrial flutter at a rate of 300 beats per minute (bpm), a dangerously rapid ventricular response could be avoided. On the other hand, a sudden drop in heart rate often is accompanied by a feeling of marked distress by the patient, especially if the rise in sinus rate occurs as a normal physiologic response to exercise. For example, a patient with an upper rate limit of 140 bpm who was jogging and developed a sinus rate above 140 bpm would abruptly develop a ventricular response of 70 bpm. This particular area of DDD pacing is one of the most complex. Programs can be devised to develop a Wenckebach phenomenon at the upper rate limit to reduce the abrupt drop in heart rate.

The upper rate limit is affected by the total atrial refractory period (TARP). TARP is defined as the AV interval plus the postventricular atrial refractory period (PVARP): TARP = AV interval + PVARP. This concept is critically important but basically can be summarized by the fact that the atrial rate can speed up to a sufficient degree that the atrial beats are no longer sensed because they fall into the atrial refractory interval (there must be a period in which there is no sensing in the atrium because of the QRS complex and also the need to reduce PMT). The upper rate limit cannot be above a certain level, depending on the TARP. This is defined in the following manner. The rate at which 2:1 block occurs is equal to 60,000 (the number of milliseconds in a minute) divided by the TARP (in msec):

$$\text{2:1 rate} = 60,000 \ (\text{msec/minute})/\text{TARP (msec)}$$

If the upper rate limit is programmed in below the 2:1 rate, the Wenckebach phenomenon can occur. If the upper rate limit is programmed greater than the

2:1 rate, then 2:1 block will occur, which may lead to patient discomfort and abrupt changes in the patient's cardiac output and blood pressure when the 2:1 block occurs. In addition to these two mechanisms of "block" at a patient's upper rate limit, some dual-chamber pacemakers can be programmed to gradually "smooth" a patient's heart rate down when the atrial rate meets or exceeds the preprogrammed 2:1 block. This is done by having the pacemaker sense that the interval of the 2:1 block has been reached. It then begins to provide a gradually slower AV synchronous pacing based on a percentage of the patient's preceding cardiac intervals. For example, if the interval the generator is using for rate smoothing is the RR interval, and if the maximum RR interval allowed is 500 msec (120 bpm) with a rate smoothing of 10%, then the next paced RR interval will be 550 msec (500 + 500 × 0.1) (109 bpm), with the atrial paced beat occurring at its preprogrammed AV interval. The next RR interval would occur at 605 msec (550 + 550 × 0.1) (99 bpm) until a slower intrinsic atrial rate is sensed or until the original targeted 2:1 rate is reached.

Automatic Mode Switching

A significant limitation to the first dual-chamber pacemakers was the presence of paroxysmal atrial tachyarrhythmias. The atrial chamber would sense the tachyarrhythmias and subsequently trigger a rapid rate and the ventricular response in a physiologically inappropriate manner. Current dual-chamber pacemakers contain sophisticated algorithms (that can be programmed to noninvasively) to sense an inappropriate rapid atrial rate and cause the dual-chamber pacemaker to switch from an atrial tracking to an atrial nontracking mode with a backup rhythm; this occurs automatically. The programming of these devices is sophisticated and allows for gradual increases and decreases in the ventricular rate to improve patient comfort. This "rate-smoothing" aspect in the presence of automatic mode switching can lead to confusing rhythm strips.

Rate-responsive AV Delay

When a patient's heart rate increases in response to exercise, for example, the normal physiologic response is to shorten the PR interval. This response maintains an appropriate PR interval at rapid heart rates. Some dual-chamber pacemakers have programs within them to mimic this behavior; this is particularly valuable in a patient with a relatively high maximum tracking rate or a maximum high sensing rate. These features can be programmable.

PROGRAMMABILITY

The presence of two pacing systems that must interact with each other increases the complexity of the programmable features of the pacemaker. These features are summarized in Table 6-1.

TABLE 6-1. *Some possible programmable features of dual-chamber pacemakers*

1. Mode of pacing (e.g., DDD, VDD, DVI, VVI, VOO, DDI, VDI)
2. AV interval (time from the atrial spike to the ventricular spike) (typical range, 80–250 msec)
3. Rate
   a. If DDD or VDD pacing is used, the ventricular rate is dependent on the patient's atrial rate. *Lower rate limit* can be programmed to control the rate at which AV sequential pacing will occur during episodes of bradycardia; (typical range, 40–80 bpm). *Upper rate limit* can be programmed to limit the maximum ventricular rate allowable in response to a supraventricular tachycardia (typical range, 100–180 bpm)
   b. If DVI or VVI pacing is used, the pacing rate is programmed routinely (typical range, 40–130 bpm)
4. Atrial pulse width
5. Atrial sensitivity
6. AV interval programmability
7. Atrial refractory period (This programmable function can be useful in eliminating endless loop tachycardia.)
   a. Atrial refractory period after sensed P-wave or atrial paced beat
   b. Post-PVC atrial refractory period extension
8. Ventricular pulse width
9. Ventricular sensitivity
10. Ventricular refractory period
11. Hysteresis
12. Rate modulating
13. Rate smoothing

AV, atrioventricular; PVC, premature ventricular contraction.

TWO CAVEATS

1. Although we have attempted to give a reasonable overview of the more complex pacemakers, the area is changing rapidly, and much of what is reviewed may soon be outdated.

2. The technology, the electrophysiology, and the follow-up of advanced-function pacemakers are more complex than we have described. Physicians recommending or implanting dual-chamber pacemakers must not only have the technical skill for the procedure but also must be sure that patient follow-up is conducted by someone who understands the technical function of the pacemaker and is capable of diagnosing and dealing with complex pacemaker arrhythmias.

TEMPORARY PACEMAKERS

Dual-chamber pacing is available with temporary pacemakers. The most common application is after open heart surgery in which the surgeon has left removable transthoracic leads to both the atrium and ventricle, and AV sequential pacing can be effected with an external pacemaker. Transvenous dual-chamber temporary pacing leads are commercially available but infrequently used.

REFERENCES

Alt EU, Von Bibra H, Blomer H. Different beneficial AV intervals with DDD pacing after sensed or paced atrial events. *J Electrophysiol* 1987;1:250.

Anderson HR, Nielsen JC. Long-term follow-up of patients from a randomised trial of atrial versus ventricular pacing for sick-sinus syndrome. *Lancet* 1997;350:1210.

Baig MW, Perrins EJ. The hemodynamics of cardiac pacing: clinical and physiological aspects. *Prog Cardiovasc Dis* 1991;33:283.

Barold S. Sustained inhibition of a DDD pacemaker at rates below the programmed lower rate during automatic PVARP extension. *Pacing Clin Electrophysiol* 1999;22:521.

Barold SS. Management of patients with dual chamber pulse generators: central role of the pacemaker atrial refractory period. *Am Coll Cardiol Highlights* 1990;5:8.

Byrd CL, Scala G, Schwartz SJ, et al. Retrograde conduction and rate responsive pacemakers. *Pacing Clin Electrophysiol* 1987;10:1208(abst).

Byrd CL, Schwartz SJ, Gonzales M, et al. DDD pacemakers maximize hemodynamic benefits and minimize complications for most patients (Part II). *Pacing Clin Electrophysiol* 1988;11:1911.

Calkins H, El-Atassi R, Kalbfleisch S, et al. Comparison of fixed burst versus decremental burst pacing for termination of ventricular tachycardia (Part I). *Pacing Clin Electrophysiol* 1993;16:26.

Chirife R, Ortega DF, Salazar AI. Nonphysiological left heart AV intervals as a result of DDD and AAI "physiological" pacing (Part II). *Pacing Clin Electrophysiol* 1991;14:1752.

Cunningham TM. Pacemaker syndrome due to retrograde conduction in a DDI pacemaker. *Am Heart J* 1988;115:478.

Dritsas A, Joshi J, Webb SC, et al. Beat-to-beat variability in stroke volume during VVI pacing as predictor of hemodynamic benefit from DDD pacing. *Pacing Clin Electrophysiol* 1993;6:1713.

Fananapazir L, Cannon RO III, Tripodi D, Panza JA. Impact of dual-chamber permanent pacing in patients with obstructive hypertrophic cardiomyopathy with symptoms refractory to verapamil and beta-adrenergic blocker therapy. *Circulation* 1992;85:2149.

Janosik DL, Pearson AC, Buckingham TA, et al. The hemodynamic benefit of differential atrioventricular delay intervals for sensed and paced atrial events during physiologic pacing. *J Am Coll Cardiol* 1989;14:499.

Jeanrenaud X, Goy J-J, Kappenberger L. Effects of dual-chamber pacing in hypertrophic obstructive cardiomyopathy. *Lancet* 1992;339:1318.

Kamalvand K, Tan K, Kotsakis A, Bucknall C, Sulke N. Is mode switching beneficial? A randomized study in patients with paroxysmal atrial tachyarrhythmias. *J Am Coll Cardiol* 1997;30:496.

Kratz J, Tyler J. Clinical experience with a new DDD external pacemaker. *Pacing Clin Electrophysiol* 1993;16:2227.

Lamas G, Orav J, Stambler B, et al. Quality of life and clinical outcomes in elderly patients treated with ventricular pacing as compared with dual-chamber pacing. *N Engl J Med* 1998;338:1097.

Leclercq C, Cazeau S, Le Breton H, et al. Acute hemodynamic effects of biventricular DDD pacing in patients with end-stage heart failure. *J Am Coll Cardiol* 1998;32:1825.

Mason J, Hlatky M. Do patients prefer physiologic pacing? *N Engl J Med* 1998;338:1147.

Mayumi H, Uchida T, Shinozaki K, Matsui K. Use of a dual chamber pacemaker with a novel fallback algorithm as an effective treatment for sick sinus syndrome associated with transient supraventricular tachyarrhythmia (Part I). *Pacing Clin Electrophysiol* 1993;16:992.

Mond HG, Barold SS. Dual chamber, rate adaptive pacing in patients with paroxysmal supraventricular tachyarrhythmias: protective measures for rate control. *Pacing Clin Electrophysiol* 1993;16:2168.

Pieterse M, Den Dulk K, Van Gelder B, Van Mechelen R, Wellens H. Programming a long paced atrioventricular interval may be risky in DDDR pacing. *Pacing Clin Electrophysiol* 1994;17:252.

Provenier F, Boudrez H, Deharo J, Djiane P, Jordaens L. Quality of life in patients with complete heart block and paroxysmal atrial tachyarrhythmias: a comparison of permanent DDIR versus DDDR pacing with mode switch to DDIR. *Pacing Clin Electrophysiol* 1999;22:462.

Ryden L. Atrial inhibited pacing—an underused mode of cardiac stimulation. *Pacing Clin Electrophysiol* 1988;11:1375.

Stroobandt R, Vandenbulcke F, Falleyn H, Sinnaeve A. Voltage dip in pacemaker battery supply: a new cause of pacemaker mediated tachycardia (Part I). *Pacing Clin Electrophysiol* 1993;16:806.

Sutton R, Stack Z, Heaven D, Ingram A. Mode switching for atrial tachyarrhythmias. *Am J Cardiol* 1999;83:202D.

7

Rate-modulated Pacing

The concept of rate-modulated (rate-responsive, rate-adaptive) pacemakers was developed to help a patient adapt to physiologic stress with an increase in heart rate, even if the patient's intrinsic sinus node normally would not allow this to occur. This step, of course, is beyond simple backup pacing for bradycardias. The development of dual-chamber pacemakers allows a patient to increase heart rate if he or she is in sinus rhythm. Many patients, however, have chronic atrial fibrillation or sick sinus syndrome that prevents normal physiologic sinus node response to exercise or stress.

Tremendous gains were made in this area during the 1980s. The approach to rate-modulated pacing can be thought of as having three components:

1. An indicator, such as activity, body temperature, or respiratory rate, that is an approximate measurement of metabolic needs
2. A sensor that can measure the indicator chosen, such as measurement of body temperature or respiratory rate
3. A rate-controlled algorithm that is in the software of the pacemaker and modulates the pacemaker rate as the sensors send signals to the pacemaker (Fig. 7-1).

INDICATORS

Vibration Sensor

A *piezoelectrode* is a quartzlike substance that, when bent, generates electric energy. A flat sheet of piezoelectric material can be placed inside the pacemaker generator. Changes in body movement and muscle motion will cause deformation of the piezoelectrode crystal. That mechanical signal is transferred to an electric signal that is, in turn, routed through sensors, filters, and other electric components, causing the pacemaker to increase or decrease its rate, depending on the amount of activity or motion sensed. A lower rate limit is set in this type of pacemaker to allow a reasonable baseline rate when no activity is sensed. A maximum rate is set for when the pacemaker is sensing considerable motion. A

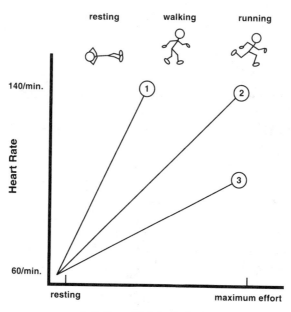

FIG. 7-1. In this example, the metabolic indicators on the horizontal axis could represent any of the indicators (e.g., body temperature or respiratory rate). The heart rate response in this example varies from 60 to 140 bpm. The sensitivity to the indicator can be programmed noninvasively. The first line would be overly sensitive, with a maximum heart rate achieved with simple walking; the next line would be ideal; and the third line would be insensitive, with a maximum heart rate not achieved even at maximal exercise. This is an idealized version, and the line actually may tend to be logarithmic or exponential. Ideally, it should be fairly linear to avoid the heart rate jumping with minimal exercise or the heart rate not becoming elevated until reaching maximal exercise.

graded ramp is incorporated into the pacemaker software for increased pacemaker rate as increased motion is recognized.

The advantages of this approach are that (a) it is a relatively simple application, (b) it does not require a special lead, (c) it is relatively sensitive, and (d) it detects motion easily. There is relatively little energy drain with this approach.

Potential disadvantages of this approach include both false-positives and false-negatives. For example, a patient standing still on a moving bus may tend to trigger the motion sensor even though there is no increased physiologic need for a higher heart rate. Conversely, a patient actively riding a bicycle on a smooth road may not trigger the sensor enough to increase the heart rate appropriately. Emotional stress would not be recognized if not accompanied by motion.

Accelerometer Motion Sensor

An *accelerometer* is a small device that can be put in the pacemaker. It differs from a piezoelectrode in that acceleration or deceleration is recognized physically by a small mass in the pacemaker, and these changes are transformed into an electric signal that is processed to increase the rate as appropriate. Accelerometers sense motion rather than vibration and can therefore have a more accurate relationship to body motion.

The accelerometer is a small weight (mass) suspended by wires tied to a frame. When the body (in the frame) moves, the mass remains still until the wires stretch and exert force causing the mass to move, allowing acceleration or deceleration to be transmitted into an electric signal.

The use of the accelerometer is fairly simple and inexpensive and is much less likely to lead to an inappropriate rise in heart rate in a situation of vibration, such as a bumpy automobile ride, using power tools, or coughing.

Temperature

At the initiation of exercise, a person's central venous pressure has a slight but abrupt drop as cooler peripheral blood is shunted into the central venous system. With further exercise, the temperature gradually rises as the metabolic rate increases. A temperature-sensing lead can be incorporated into the pacemaker lead, and the pacemaker can respond to temperature changes. Available thermistors are capable of detecting minute temperature changes, and this appears to be a reliable mode of rate-response pacing. If a patient has a fever, the temperature is monitored over the long term, and appropriate adjustments are made so that the fever does not result in extremely rapid pacing over the long term.

An advantage of using body temperature as an indicator includes its accuracy as a reasonable estimate of metabolic need. One potential disadvantage is that it requires a "dedicated lead" for a specific use and, if changes are contemplated in the future or if this approach were abandoned at some point in the future, a new lead would need to be placed.

One concern that has often been raised is if the patient develops a fever. In general, the sensor will note a prolonged temperature rise that plateaus and will allow the heart rate to drop to a reasonable rate so that this does not represent a risk to the patient.

This sensor has been on the market in the past but has not gained widespread acceptance.

Catecholamines

Serum catecholamines increase with activity, but direct measurement is not readily feasible. Catecholamines increase the contractility of the heart and shorten the QT interval, even if the heart rate is fixed. QT interval sensors that detect the time interval between a ventricular QRS complex and the peak of the T wave are currently fairly accurate. As emotional or physical stress occurs, the catecholamine present shortens the QT interval, and sensors are capable of noting this change and adjusting the patient rate accordingly. This type of pacemaker may need reprogramming because of changes related to electrolytes, medications, ischemia, and hypertrophy. A similar approach includes measurement of the area under the QRS complex. Catecholamines shorten the QRS complex somewhat. This approach is under investigation as a sensor similar to the QT interval.

Increased catecholamine stimulation reduces the preejection period, which is measured from the onset of the QRS complex to the beginning of mechanical systole. Devices that can measure stroke volume through impedance measurements as described in Figure 7-2 can use the preejection period as a metabolic indicator.

Right Ventricular Stroke Volume

Relative stroke volume can be estimated fairly accurately through impedance measurements similar to the concept illustrated in Figure 7-2. With diastole, there is more electrolyte solution for electricity to pass through and impedance is lower. With systole, there is less electrolyte solution in the right ventricle and impedance is higher. This is a somewhat complex measurement and has generally not received commercial acceptance.

Right Ventricular Pressure

Right ventricular pressure with dP/dT (change in pressure over time) measurement is a physiologic indicator that can be measured with a dedicated lead. This involves pressure monitors placed at the tip of the lead and has not yet been developed as a commercially available, long-term, stable approach.

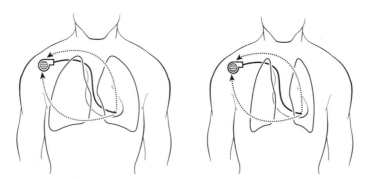

FIG. 7-2. Minute ventilation is measured by frequent tiny electric signals placed during the respiratory cycle. The small electric signal is between the lead tip and the pacemaker generator. Because there is a known voltage, the current can be measured and the resistance (or impedence) calculated. During inspiration, the impedence is relatively high because there is more air and less electrolyte solution for electricity to pass through. During expiration, the impedence is relatively low because there is less air and more electrolyte solution. Although these differences are quite small, they can be measured accurately, and minute ventilation can be estimated with a high degree of reproducibility and accuracy.

Minute Ventilation (Respiration)

Respiration sensors are available for physiologic pacing and represent a fairly good measurement of metabolic need related to activity or stress. One approach to measurement of respiratory rate would be measuring diaphragmatic motion with intrapleural pressure measurement. Deflection of a piezoelectrode could generate an electric signal indicating a respiratory change. The more common method for measuring respiratory rate uses the fact that transthoracic impedance changes with the respiration. The impedance between a pacemaker generator and a reference electrode (see Fig. 7-2) changes with respiratory rates. As the lungs inflate with inspiration, there will be higher resistance, which can be detected by the impedance sensor.

Measurement of changes in impedance can be used to estimate minute ventilation, and pacemaker rate can change appropriately. Having a rate-adaptive pacemaker respond to minute ventilation may have advantages over response to respiratory rate. For example, with exertion minute ventilation will increase, but if the patient hyperventilates without exertion, respiratory rate will go up, but often total volume will go down and minute ventilation may remain close to baseline.

Compared with motion sensors, the minute ventilation is a somewhat slower response to activity. It may, however, shorten the battery life by approximately 1 year in some systems. The frequent spikes can interfere with the electrocardiogram (EKG) (Fig. 7-3), especially transtelephonic measurements, which may accentuate the spikes.

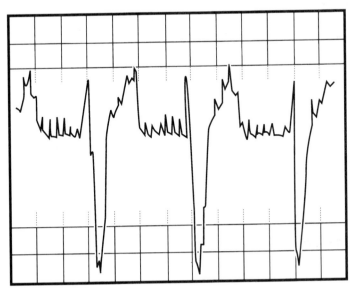

FIG. 7-3. This rhythm strip was taken from a patient with a minute ventilation sensor. In this particular patient, the spikes placed by the pacemaker during the respiratory cycle can be seen on the rhythm strip. In other leads, with a different axis, however, they may be invisible. A transtelephonic pacemaker checking device may be particularly susceptible to this type of interference because the spikes are artificially accentuated.

pH Measurements

During exercise, pH of the venous blood decreases with lactic acid production; pH sensors are available but have not demonstrated long-term stability.

Central Oxygen Saturation

Central oxygen saturation of the right ventricle also could be used with a lead in the right ventricle and a measuring system of oxygen saturation, which is an accurate metabolic indicator; however, the technology available to measure this with long-term stability is somewhat problematic.

Combined Sensor Utilization

The combination of activity sensors, which are relatively inexpensive, with another sensor, such as the minute ventilation, is now available. Some of the advantages of the sensors can be combined this way.

RATE–RESPONSE ALGORITHM

The pacemaker must convert any sensed activity or metabolic indicator into an appropriate rate. This concept is presented in Figure 7-1. Basically, the sensor, whether it be body motion, temperature, or respiratory rate, is on the horizontal axis. As the sensor indicates greater metabolic need, the pacemaker software causes the patient's rate to increase. Three different "ramps" are demonstrated. The first represents an overly sensitive setting in which the patient develops a high heart rate with minimal exercise (e.g., walking). The second represents an ideal approach in which the heart rate increases in response to metabolic need during activity. The third represents a possibly overly dampened response in which the patient never can develop a particularly elevated heart rate despite vigorous activity. These represent idealized ramps. Often the ramp has a curve, either upward or downward. The nature of the curve needs to be considered and can lead to an inappropriately sensitive or insensitive response to metabolic need. This is an engineering problem that will be determined by individual pacemaker manufacturers.

After implantation of a rate-modulated pacemaker, ideally the patient should undergo exercise or ambulatory heart-rate monitoring or both to assess the heart rate response to the indicator used. This area tends to be neglected.

The initial rate—response pacemakers available have been placed on VVI pacemakers because the technology is less complex. Now DDDR pacemakers are becoming available, increasing the complexity of the dual-chamber pacemakers considerably. One intuitive outcome of this may be that there could be an element of "rate smoothing" at the upper limit of the DDD pacemaker. The pacemaker may develop heart block in relation to the normal sinus rhythm at peak exercise, but the sensor may overdrive any heart block (e.g., Wenckebach or 2:1 block occurring at the upper rate limit of the pacemaker) and lead to atrial pacing at a faster rate, which is sensor driven rather than driven by the patient's intrinsic sinus rhythm.

Rate-modulated pacing may open up further approaches, but these are not well established. For instance, DDIR and DVIR modes may be used in patients with dual-chamber pacemakers who are active but who also have sinus node dysfunction with questionable AV conduction and undesirable atrial arrhythmias. This type of programming would not track undesirable atrial arrhythmias (e.g., rapid atrial flutter or atrial fibrillation) but would maintain many of the other beneficial aspects of AV sequential pacing and rate-responsive pacing.

Once again, however, if the patient has an intact sinus node and intact sinus node function with exercise, the sinus rate will increase appropriately, and a DDD AV sequential pacemaker would be the simplest form of rate-modulated pacing. Some companies are working with dual-sensor technology, with two different types of sensing leading to rate-modulated pacing. Dual sensing, however, introduces a significant element of complexity for the clinician.

RATE-MODULATED TEMPORARY PACING

A rate-modulated temporary pacemaker is not available and is not required. Patients with temporary pacemakers are generally on bed rest, and rates can be changed easily by using the temporary pacemaker, depending on metabolic and electrophysiologic needs.

REFERENCES

Abrahamsen AM, Barvik S, Aarsland T, Dickstein K. Rate responsive cardiac pacing using a minute ventilation sensor. *Pacing Clin Electrophysiol* 1993;16:1650.

Alt E. What is the ideal rate-adaptive sensor for patients with implantable cardioverter defibrillators: lessons from cardiac pacing. *Am J Cardiol* 1999;83:17D.

Bacharach D, Hilden T, Millerhagen J, Westrum B, Kelly J. Activity-based pacing: comparison of a device using an accelerometer versus a piezoelectric crystal. *Pacing Clin Electrophysiol* 1992;15:188.

Brandt J, Fahraeus T, Ogawa T, Schuller H. Practical aspects of rate adaptive atrial (AAI,R) pacing: clinical experiences in 44 patients. *Pacing Clin Electrophysiol* 1991;14:1258.

Candinas R, Jakob M, Buckingham T, Mattmann H, Amann F. Vibration, acceleration, gravitation, and movement: activity controlled rate adaptive pacing during treadmill exercise testing and daily life activities. *Pacing Clin Electrophysiol* 1997;20:1777.

Chirife R, Ortega DF, Salazar AI. Feasibility of measuring relative right ventricular volumes and ejection fraction with implantable rhythm control devices. *Pacing Clin Electrophysiol* 1993;16:1673.

Clementy J, Barold S, Garrigue S, et al. Clinical significance of multiple sensor options: rate response optimization, sensor blending, and trending. *Am J Cardiol* 1999;83:166D.

Connelly DT. The Topaz Study Group: initial experience with a new single chamber, dual sensor rate responsive pacemaker. *Pacing Clin Electrophysiol* 1993;16:1833.

Cowell R, Morris-Thurgood J, Paul V, et al. Are we being driven to two sensors? Clinical benefits of sensor cross-checking. *Pacing Clin Electrophysiol* 1993;16:1441.

Lamas GA, Keefe JM. The effects of equitation (horseback riding) on a motion responsive DDDR pacemaker (Part I). *Pacing Clin Electrophysiol* 1990;13:1371.

Landzberg J, Franklin J, Mahawar S, et al. Benefits of physiologic atrioventricular synchronization for pacing with an exercise rate response. *Am J Cardiol* 1990;66:193.

Mond H, Barold S. Dual chamber, rate adaptive pacing in patients with paroxysmal supraventricular tach-yarrhythmias: protective measures for rate control. *Pacing Clin Electrophysiol* 1993;16:2168.

Mond H, Strathmore N, Kertes P, et al. Rate responsive pacing using a minute ventilation sensor (Part II). *PACE* 1988;11:1866.

Oda E. Changes in QT interval during exercise testing in patients with VVI pacemakers (Part I). *Pacing Clin Electrophysiol* 1986;9:36.

Sellers TD, Fearnot NE, Smith HJ, et al. Right ventricular blood temperature profiles for rate responsive pacing (Part I). *Pacing Clin Electrophysiol* 1987;10:467.

Sulke N, Chambers J, Dritsas A, Sowton E. A randomized double-blind crossover comparison of four rate-responsive pacing modes. *J Am Coll Cardiol* 1991;17:696.

Vanerio G, Maloney JD, Pinski SL, et al. DDIR versus VVIR pacing in patients with paroxysmal atrial tachyarrhythmias (Part I). *Pacing Clin Electrophysiol* 1991;14:1630.

Vanerio G, Patel S, Ching E, et al. Early clinical experience with a minute ventilation sensor DDDR pace-maker (Part II). *Pacing Clin Electrophysiol* 1991;14:1815.

8

Implantable Cardioverter Defibrillator and Antitachycardia Pacing

The implantable cardioverter defibrillator (ICD), an electric device similar to the pacemaker, has undergone revolutionary changes in the last 5 years. Originally called an *automatic implantable cardioverter-defibrillator* (AICD) when only one company marketed the device, the abbreviation *ICD* now is used as a generic term for implantable defibrillators produced by all companies. Although the device initially was developed only to defibrillate patients with ventricular tachycardia or ventricular fibrillation who did not respond to antiarrhythmic drug therapy, the more recent models are able to provide low-energy cardioversion, antitachycardia pacing termination, and bradycardia pacing backup.

The idea for a fully implantable, automatic device for the recognition of ventricular arrhythmias was proposed by Mirowski in 1981. An ICD is similar to a pacemaker in that it also is an electric circuit requiring a closed loop. In the ICD, electricity is directed across a large portion of the myocardium to depolarize most of the ventricle, thereby allowing an organized rhythm to return.

INDICATIONS

Determining who is a candidate for an ICD usually involves a thorough evaluation by a cardiac electrophysiologist. Complete testing may include an echocardiogram, evaluation of ejection fraction, cardiac catheterization, electrophysiologic testing, possible serial drug testing, exercise test, ambulatory monitoring, signal averaged electrocardiogram (ECG), and evaluation of the need for a permanent pacemaker. As with any novel therapy, the indications for the ICD are evolving. In the past, the ICD was used for patients who had survived a sudden cardiac death event or had been identified as being at extremely high risk. More recently, however, indications have been expanded to include those who have had asymptomatic nonsustained ventricular tachycardia with decreased ventricular function.

The type of internal defibrillator used, including the type of backup ventricular pacemaker (dual-chamber or single chamber), is selected according to the clinical needs.

Contraindications to pacemaker placement include a reversible cause to the cardiac arrest (such as acute myocardial ischemia), atrial fibrillation with a rapid ventricular response (which may occur as a result of a bypass tract as in Wolff–Parkinson–White syndrome), or electrolyte abnormalities. Associated illnesses with an expected short-term survival also would be a contraindication. With the foreign body, active septicemia would be a contraindication.

Specific indications for ICD therapy include the following:

1. Cardiac arrest not attributable to transient or irreversible etiology
2. Known sustained ventricular tachycardia
3. Syncope of undetermined etiology with a positive electrophysiologic study for inducible ventricular tachycardia or ventricular fibrillation
4. Nonsustained ventricular tachycardia with underlying coronary artery disease with prior myocardial infarction or left ventricular dysfunction with inducible ventricular tachycardia or ventricular fibrillation during electrophysiologic study, not suppressible by antiarrhythmic therapy
5. Symptomatic ventricular tachycardia with a defibrillator to be used as a bridge to cardiac transplantation
6. Inherited long QT syndrome or hypertrophic cardiomyopathy with high risk for sudden cardiac death

GENERATOR

The size of the generator required for the ICD varies between less than 40 to 60 cc. These generators are similar in size to the original pacemakers and now can be placed within the chest wall (the original ones could be placed only within the abdominal wall because of their size). The largest component of the generator is the capacitor. There is ongoing research to miniaturize capacitors. ICDs will be placed in the pectoral region, allowing the procedure to be performed in the catheterization laboratory. Such a device would need to have a volume of less than 100 cc and be 25 mm thick.

The battery used in the ICD is usually the lithium silver vanadium oxide, which allows rapid discharge into a capacitor for the frequent rapid shocks that may be required of the ICD device. The capacitor and batteries together account for 75% to 80% of the generator's volume. Longevity is currently estimated to be 4 to 10 years, depending on the frequency of use.

LEADS

A simplified picture of the AICD lead is shown in Figure 8-1. The leads are available for rate sensing, pacing, and shocking.

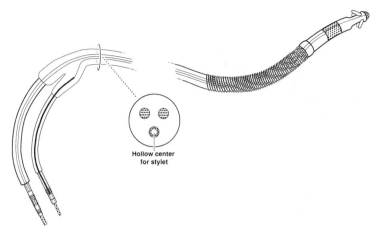

Hollow center
for stylet

FIG. 8-1. Automatic implantable cardioverter–defibrillator (*ICD*). This is a schematic diagram of cardioverter–defibrillation lead. The stippled areas, as in most pictures in this text, represent exposed metal. The distal two areas of exposed metal of the lead represent the bipolar pacemaker. There is a tip and band electrode, as in a typical bipolar pacemaker. The more proximal larger exposed metal is a coiled metal band that is one pole of the defibrillator. This connects back up to the defibrillator generator. A comparatively large charge of electricity can flow between this pole and the wall of the defibrillator itself, which represents the other pole (through an internal connection to the defibrillator battery). The leads are encased in silicone and separated from each other. One of the pacemaker leads will have a hollow center to allow for a stiffer stylet to be placed through to assist the clinician in placing the lead transvenously.

The lead shown would be placed in the right ventricle, which would provide continuous sensing of the ventricular rate and the fundamental criteria and for detection of sustained ventricular tachyarrhythmias. The current systems incorporate both therapy and rate-sensing function to a single transvenous endocardial lead for simplicity. The bipolar lead can pace in the ventricle and sense the ventricular rate, and the shocking portion of the lead can provide a large electric charge between the coil and pacing lead.

For the sake of simplicity, we have not shown the more complex systems that also incorporate an atrial lead. The atrial lead can be used to count atrial beats (the comparison of atrial beats in relation to ventricular beats can be helpful in deciding whether a rhythm is ventricular tachycardia or supraventricular tachycardia). For instance, with ventricular tachycardia and complete atrioventricular (AV) disassociation, the atrial rate would be much lower than the ventricular rate. If the patient is in supraventricular tachycardia with 1:1 or 1:2 conduction, that information may be useful in determining the exact nature of the arrhythmia. This is a complex area and requires an electrophysiologist to make programming decisions.

BASIC SYSTEM OPERATION

The operation of the ICD is similar to that of the pacemaker in that the two basic functions are sensing and delivering electricity. ICDs can be traced back through three generations of development. The first devices could detect ventricular tacycardia (VT) or ventricular fibrillation (VF) and, after a certain elapsed period, charge the capacitor and deliver a nonprogrammable, nonsynchronized shock of 25 to 30 joules (J), up to a maximum of five consecutive times unless the tachycardia was terminated. The second generation of devices provided programmable low-energy cardioversion in addition to the conventional high-energy shocks. The third and present generation of ICDs feature what is referred to as *tiered therapy*, which includes antitachycardia pacing for painless termination of monomorphic VT, programmable low-energy cardioversion, high-energy defibrillation, and backup bradycardia pacing. Figure 8-2 demon-

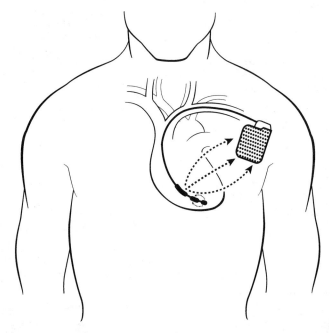

FIG. 8-2. In this schematic demonstration of a single-lead pacing defibrillator device, the *solid arrows* demonstrate a shock with electricity flowing between the large proximal band and the wall of the can, which represents the other pole. The generator is usually placed in the left anterior chest, which allows more of the electricity to go through the left ventricle in an effort to defibrillate it. The tip and band electrode of the bipolar pacemaker are shown with a separate electric current available for pacing (of course, the shock and the pacing will not be simultaneous). This is shown schematically for simplification. Fig. 8-1 shows a more detailed view of the lead. Also, commonly dual-chamber pacemakers are used to pace in both the atrium and ventricle. This is not shown again for simplicity's sake. The addition of an atrial lead, however, allows not only pacing of the atrium but also sensing of atrial activity to improve the accuracy of diagnosis of ventricular tachycardia as opposed to supraventricular tachycardia.

strates the concept of the shocking and pacing. The large proximal electrode is one pole, and the metallic covering of the generator is the other pole. This represents the large shock for defibrillation or cardioversion from rapid tachycardia. The tip and band electrode of the typical pacing lead are shown with small dots indicating the potential for pacing (of course, they would not be pacing and shocking at the same time).

In addition, they have the ability to perform noninvasive electrophysiologic (EP) testing and are able to store electrograms after a shock has occurred, therefore assisting the physician in identifying types and numbers of therapies delivered when the patient returns for checkups. The tiered therapy devices have proven beneficial and more acceptable in patients who can be converted out of their tachycardia by painless pacing or low-level cardioversion rather than the more painful defibrillation. In a tiered device, however, if the tachycardia is not converted with these lower-energy therapies after a preprogrammed period, defibrillation is initiated.

TACHYCARDIA DETECTION

The fundamental way the ICD identifies the presence of a sustained ventricular tachyarrhythmia is by detecting that heart rate has exceeded a critical value. Because most episodes of sustained VT exhibit a rate in excess of 150 beats per minute (bpm), the device can be programmed to initiate therapy when this rate is reached. The type of therapy to be used depends on the device as well as the hemodynamic status of the patient during the tachyarrhythmia episode. For antitachycardia pacing, additional detection criteria may be programmed to enhance the certainty that a ventricular tachyarrhythmia is present rather than a supraventricular tachyarrhythmia (SVT), usually atrial fibrillation. Such "detection enhancements" include the identification of cycle length stability, the abruptness of onset of the tachyarrhythmia, and the duration of a sustained rate. Attempts to measure the electrogram with the criteria have been somewhat less successful in sorting out VT from SVT. Because VF often manifests as rates in excess of 240 bpm, the ICD is usually programmed to respond to such rates by defibrillation. With tiered therapy devices, rate ranges can be programmed that determine the type of therapy to be delivered. Thus, with rates of 150 to 230 bpm, antitachycardia pacing or low-energy cardioversion can be used; for rates greater than 230 bpm, defibrillation is the programmed response. The cutoff values for rate that dictate the type of therapy can be tailored to the individual patient.

As mentioned, the dual-chamber ICD will allow counting of atrial rates in comparison to ventricular rates. For instance, if the ventricular rate is greater than the atrial rate, the ICD can be programmed to treat (again this requires an electrophysiologist; for example, because of the risk of ventricular tachycardia leading to retrograde AV conduction and 1:1 relation of ventricular and atrial rates).

THERAPY TIERS

Bradycardia Pacing

As indicated, about 10% of patients successfully converted out of VT or VF are found to have marked sinus bradycardia immediately postconversion, posing another threat to hemodynamic stability. Therefore, modern ICD devices often have the option of VVI pacing, DDD pacing, DDDR pacing, AAI pacing, and AAIR pacing. After a shock, there may be an increased threshold required to pace. Therefore, as a precaution, a higher output can be programmed for several beats after the shock.

Antitachycardia Pacing

Many episodes of VT are amenable to termination by a technique known as *overdrive pacing*, which is based on the observation that the mechanism of VT involves reentry, a circulating wavefront of excitation within a discrete region of myocardium. Between the leading edge of the wavefront and the tail of refractoriness, just ahead of the circulating wavefront is a region known as the *excitable gap*, which represents a segment of excitable myocardial tissue about to be depolarized by the propagating wavefront; thus, it "circulates" with the wave of excitation. If a critically timed premature impulse (or train of paced impulses) arrives at the site of reentry such that the impulse invades the circuit when the excitable gap permits, the circus movement will be terminated abruptly because of the collision of the two wavefronts (Fig. 8-3). Because a train of rapidly paced impulses increases the probability of invasion of the excitable gap, antitachycardia pacing usually uses a "burst" of ventricular paced impulses. Antitachycardia pacing usually is indicated as first-line treatment in patients with VT under 180 bpm. For some patients, this slower rate of tachycardia may be hemodynamically stable and may provide the opportunity for a form of therapy that is painless and requires lesser current drain. Therefore, pacing for termination may be effective and more desirable from a comfort standpoint. When this form of therapy is programmed, initial response to tachycardia will be a burst of pacing impulses delivered at a rapid rate. Up to 15 paced impulses per burst may be delivered at a time. Different modes of tachypacing delivery may be built into devices from different manufacturers.

Burst pacing can be programmed in one of two ways. *Ramp pacing* (Fig. 8-4A) involves delivery of impulses at successively closer intervals so that the pacing rate is actually accelerating during the burst ("within burst" decrement). *Scanning* ("between burst" decrement) involves progressively faster pacing rates with each subsequent burst (Fig. 8-4B). If the tachycardia is not successfully terminated after a predetermined number of pacing attempts, a more aggressive therapy option is activated, usually low-energy cardioversion. An example of antitachycardia pacing with successful restoration of sinus rhythm is shown in Figure 8-5A.

FIG. 8-4. Two methods of antitachycardia pacing. A: Burst pacing is illustrated using the *ramp* sequence. Note the "within burst" decrement of cycle length. B: In the *scan* sequence or "between burst" decrement, the cycle length is constant during any given burst, but it decreases progressively with each successive train.

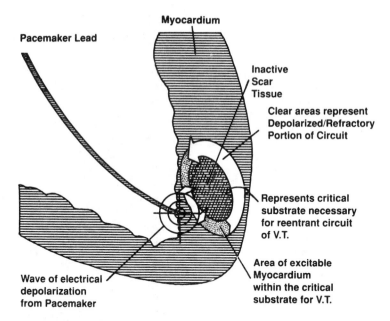

Myocardium

Pacemaker Lead

Inactive
Scar
Tissue

Clear areas represent
Depolarized/Refractory
Portion of Circuit

Represents critical
substrate necessary
for reentrant circuit
of V.T.

Area of excitable
Myocardium
within the critical
substrate for V.T.

Wave of electrical
depolarization
from Pacemaker

FIG. 8-3. A schematic, simplified representation of how tachypacing can break up a reentrant rhythm. In this example, there is an area of critical substrate necessary for the reentrant circuit of the ventricular tachycardia (VT); this is shown going in a circular area in a small portion of the myocardium, but for every circuit, electricity would exit this area and excite the entire ventricle. The pacemaker lead is able to excite a portion of that critical substrate so that when the circuit arrhythmia begins to make another circuit, it runs into depolarized tissue, and the reentrant tachycardia is stopped. This is an oversimplification. The critical substrate would rarely be right at the area of the pacemaker tip. This does, however, describe the concept in which a properly timed paced beat can break up a reentrant tachycardia and stop it.

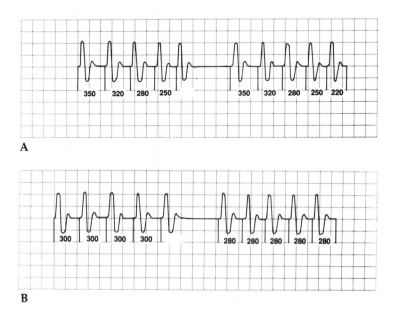

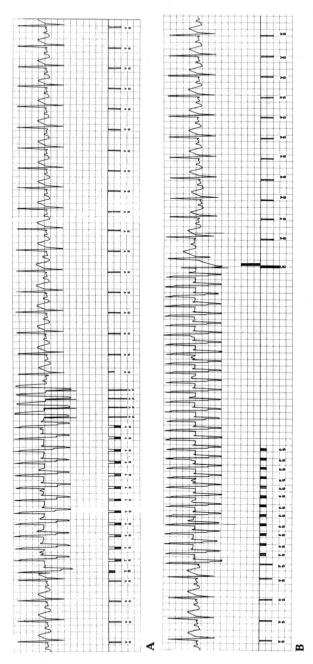

FIG. 8-5. Therapy tiers. **A:** Spontaneous ventricular tachycardia (*VT*) is detected and treated with a train of pacing stimuli at a fixed cycle length, resulting in tachycardia termination and restoration of sinus rhythm. **B:** Following tachycardia detection, therapy consists of synchronized delivery of a low-energy shock.

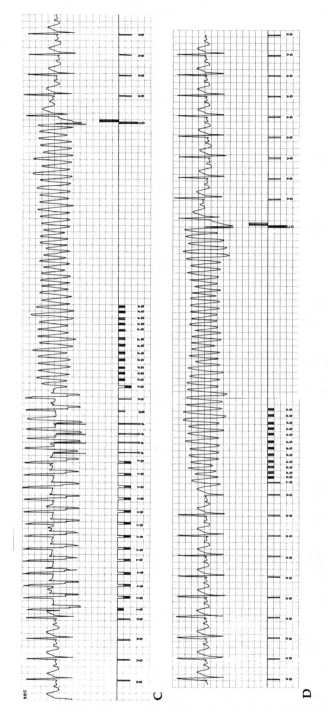

FIG. 8-5. *Continued.* **C:** Antitachycardia pacing results in tachycardia acceleration and leads to delivery of a low-energy synchronized cardioversion pulse to terminate tachycardia. **D:** Ventricular fibrillation (*VT*) is detected, and sinus rhythm is restored following a high-energy defibrillation output.

Low-energy Cardioversion

Low-level cardioversion is occasionally the first-line treatment for VT with rates greater than 180 bpm. These patients may be hemodynamically unstable and require more prompt tachycardia termination (Fig. 8-5B). The tiered ICD delivers the cardioversion synchronized with the QRS complex, thus avoiding the vulnerable period of the T wave and risking initiation of VF. The amount of energy may be programmed to a minimum of 0.1 J. Significant reduction in pain perception may be noted below 2 J, whereas no perceptible differences may be observed between 5 and 34 J in many patients. The current required for conversion will vary with electrode location and the shape and surface area of the lead system being used. Another factor in conversion success may be the direction in which electricity travels across the heart. More efficient cardioversion can be effected by improvements in lead design, lead arrangement, the pattern of energy delivery (sequential versus simultaneous), and the shape of the pulse waveform (biphasic versus monophasic). If antitachycardia pacing or cardioversion fails to terminate the tachycardia after a programmed time interval or if the tachycardia accelerates, defibrillation therapy will be initiated (Fig. 8-5C).

Defibrillation

Defibrillation is the first-line therapy when VF is the presenting rhythm. For defibrillation, electric current delivery does not need to be synchronized with a given portion of the ECG complex. After the patient has been in VF for a programmed interval, shocks that may range between 50 and 150 V or 0.1-38 J will be delivered (Fig. 8-5D). If the first shock fails to terminate the rhythm, subsequent shocks will be delivered, usually up to five or six, depending on the manufacturer and what has been programmed.

Attempts are being made to find more efficient and effective methods of shock delivery to decrease the amount of electricity needed for conversion. The success of these attempts will allow further downsizing of the generator volume and make pectoral implant more of a reality. One of these approaches has been changing the shock delivery from a unidirectional or monophasic shock waveform to bidirectional or biphasic waveforms. This is generally the standard throughout the industry at this point. Another approach to more effective defibrillation has been the delivery of pulses simultaneously over two current pathways. These changes in current delivery have been instrumental in making the transvenous lead system a reality.

USE OF MAGNETS

A magnet placed over the generator often can be used to deactivate the ICD in the event of inappropriate shocks. What a magnet does or does not do depends on the program and the manufacturer, but most commonly the magnet, while in place, will suspend the ICD therapy with no effect on pacing. Again, the electrophysiologist and the physician caring for the patient need to be aware of the clinical situation and the manufacturer's specifications so that together they may determine what programming is to be done.

DEVICE–DEVICE AND DRUG–DEVICE INTERACTIONS

Occasionally, the patient who requires a defibrillator also will require a pacemaker. As this situation becomes more frequent, more is learned about the potential interactions that can occur. One such problem is overcounting, which happens because the ICD perceives a unipolar pacing spike to be a ventricular complex. Therefore, all pacemakers implanted in ICD patients should be programmed to bipolar pacing. In addition, some pacemakers revert to a backup mode of unipolar pacing after electric shock, or some revert to a VOO mode, whether that be from the device or from externally delivered therapy. Therefore, the manufacturer's information regarding this behavior should be checked before a specific pacemaker is implanted in the ICD patient. There have also been documented accounts of defibrillator therapy being withheld during VF because of the device erroneously sensing pacemaker spikes as being QRSs.

Medical devices other than pacemakers also may interfere with ICD operation. Use of radiofrequency generators [e.g., electrocautery units used in surgery, transcutaneous electronic nerve stimulation (TENS) units, and acupuncture needles used with electrical current] all may be perceived by the ICD as the presence of ventricular rhythms. Therefore, during the use of these devices, the ICD should be programmed off or temporarily disabled using a magnet. The use of magnetic resonance imaging systems and lithotripsy devices should never be tried with ICD patients as permanent damage to the device will occur.

Magnetic devices in the environment also should be avoided by the ICD patient because these may temporarily disable the device. Magnetic devices to avoid include arc welders, stereo speakers, airport security wands (patients need to request a hand search), bingo wands, 12-V starters, industrial equipment, induction furnaces, large generators or power plants, and citizens band (CB) or ham radio antennas. Patients also should avoid touching spark plugs or distributors on running engines.

Patients with implanted ICDs may require continued antiarrhythmic medications to help control tachycardia. Initiation of new drugs or changing dosages of current medications may increase the amount of energy required to defibrillate [defibrillation threshold (DFT)]. For example, amiodarone may increase the DFT. In addition, the tachycardia morphology and rate may be altered in such a way that the originally programmed treatment protocols may no longer be effective or may shock inappropriately. It is also possible that the drug therapy itself may have a proarrhythmic effect and be responsible for initiation of a new tachycardia. Therefore, whenever changes are made in drug therapy, it is recommended that retesting and possibly reprogramming of the device take place.

HOSPITAL DISCHARGE AND DISCHARGE TESTING

Before the patient is discharged from the hospital, the ICD patient is brought back into the electrophysiology laboratory for testing of the device. With the newer ICDs, this can be performed noninvasively by using the device programmer. The programmer can be used to initiate tachycardia so that its performance can be observed in a controlled situation. Any programming changes that are required can be performed at this time. In addition, this allows the patient to experience therapy consciously in the supportive medical environment, thus reducing anxiety regarding the sensation of being defibrillated.

Discharge instructions will include avoiding lifting and contact sports, avoiding strong magnetic forces, observing the incision for signs of infection or erosion, avoiding restrictive clothing and use of an abdominal support, wearing a medical alert bracelet, and carrying a device identification card and physician letter explaining the device. The patient usually is prohibited from driving for at least 6 months and possibly indefinitely, depending on subsequent arrhythmic events, the clinician's judgment, and state laws. This issue is currently riddled with much controversy, but most electrophysiologists are taking a more liberal viewpoint than initially advanced. Patients usually are asked to report when their device fires. Families often are encouraged to learn cardiopulmonary resuscitation as a backup in the event the device fails to terminate the tachycardia.

Patients with ICDs and their families deal with many psychological issues postresuscitation and postimplantation. Independence issues surface, as do fears of death, fears of the device, major lifestyle changes, and a feeling of uncertainty about the future. Referral to psychologists and social workers often prove helpful. In addition, some medical centers offer support group meetings that give patients and their families a chance to receive further education about their device and "healthy heart living" and an opportunity to support each other through sharing of common feelings and experiences.

COMPLICATIONS AND FOLLOW-UP CARE

Complications following ICD implant are noted in up to 15% of cases, with in-hospital mortality of about 4% to 5%, generally resulting from complications of open chest surgery. In the future, the hospital mortality figures may decline with the newly available nonthoracotomy, transvenous leads. This advance opens up therapy to groups of people generally labeled poor surgical risks. Among complications of ICD therapy are ICD infections, malfunction, spurious discharges, lead fractures, pericarditis, pacemaker interaction, vein thrombosis, and "twiddler's syndrome" (pocket manipulation by the patient).

Initially, ICD patients are seen in the office 1 to 3 weeks after implantation for examination of all incision sites and assessment of device functioning. This visit is followed by office visits about every 3 months. During these visits, routine vital signs are taken and weight is measured, the heart and lungs are auscultated, and inquiry is made about any heart-related symptoms, any additions or changes in medication routine, and a history of known device discharges. The implantation site is inspected, and the device is interrogated with the programmer. Information retrieved includes the number of tachycardia detections, therapies, types and dates of therapy, and device status information, such as battery voltage, capacitor function, and current programmed values. With the newer tiered-therapy devices, information may be downloaded onto a computer disk and stored or analyzed. The stored electrograms immediately preceding and during recent detections or therapies can be replayed for verification of appropriate function.

FUTURE TRENDS

The future promises changes in every area of ICD functioning and design. New waveforms are being investigated to become more efficient and less energy consuming. The size of the ICDs continues to decrease, particularly with new research in capacitor design. Variable pathways of current delivery have become more common, and investigation continues in that area. The treatment of atrial arrhythmias (either automatic or patient activated) is being investigated. Follow-up will be enhanced by improved telecommunications, and remote follow-up will become more common. Hemodynamic sensors eventually may help to determine the type of therapy delivery. Finally, cost reduction will have to be a major goal. Although the devices remain expensive, with a longer life, the cost per year therapy is less.

TEMPORARY PACEMAKERS

The "temporary pacemaker" version of the ICD is, of course, the routine defibrillation or cardioversion used in any acute medical facility. We reiterate that there is a difference between *defibrillation* and *cardioversion*. When the device used to shock the patient is switched on defibrillation, it will shock the patient's chest when the buttons are pushed. This is necessary if the patient is in VF and there is generally nothing to "sense" and synchronize. On the other hand, if the patient were in VT rather than VF, this type of shock could end on the T wave of a QRS complex and make matters worse by converting from VT to VF.

Conversely, if cardioversion is used, the device must sense the patient's QRS complex (obviously in a full cardiac arrest with the patient in VF there is no need to make this attachment). If a patient is in VF and the device is set for cardioversion, a shock may not be delivered. If the fibrillatory waves are not sensed, the operator may keep pushing the buttons and have nothing happen and, in the confusion of a cardiac arrest, think that the machine is malfunctioning. Most of the devices we have been acquainted with tend to switch to defibrillation when the machine is first turned on because this is the emergent setting in which the machine is used, as cardioversions are usually more elective (unless the patient is hemodynamically unstable).

One development that may "spill over" from the ICD to the external defibrillator is the use of a biphasic wave form for cardioverting or defibrillating the patient. The current experience is relatively new, but some preliminary data suggest that the new waveform may be more effective.

Also, automatic external defibrillators are becoming more common in the community with lay personnel being trained in their use. This remains a somewhat controversial public health issue, but important work is being done in this area.

Temporary pacemakers for interrupting tachycardias have been available for some time. A specialized temporary pacemaker with rapid pacing rates is available. This procedure is best done by someone with sophistication in electrophysiology. Devices used in the electrophysiology laboratory provide for detailed placement of antitachycardiac pacing spikes to break up the tachyarrhythmia.

REFERENCES

Akhtar M, Jazayeri M, Sra J, et al. Implantable cardioverter defibrillator for prevention of sudden cardiac death in patients with ventricular tachycardia and ventricular fibrillation: ICD therapy in sudden cardiac death (Part II). *Pacing Clin Electrophysiol* 1993;16:511.

Almeida HF, Buckingham TA. Inappropriate implantable cardioverter defibrillator shocks secondary to sensing lead failure: utility of stored electrograms (Part I). *Pacing Clin Electrophysiol* 1993;16:407.

Ayers G, Tacker W, Gonzalez X, Schoenlein W, Janas W, Alferness C. Experience with a single pass atrial defibrillation lead system. *Circulation* 1995;92:I-472(abst).

Bardy GH, Troutman C, Poole JE, et al. Clinical experience with a tiered-therapy, multiprogrammable antiarrhythmia device. *Circulation* 1992;85:1689.

Bernstein AD, Camm AJ, Fisher JD, et al. The NASPE/BPEG defibrillator code (NASPE policy statement). *J Intervent Cardiol* 1993;6:235, and *PACE* 1993;16:1776.

Bigger JT. Prophylactic use of implanted cardiac defibrillators in patients at high risk for ventricular arrhythmias after coronary-artery bypass graft surgery. *N Engl J Med* 1997;337:1569.

Brugada J. Is inappropriate therapy a resolved issue with current implantable cardioverter defibrillators? *Am J Cardiol* 1999;83:40D.

Brugada P, Brugada R, Brugada J, Geelen P. Use of the prophylactic implantable cardioverter defibrillator for patients with normal hearts. *Am J Cardiol* 1999;83:98D.

Calkins H, Brinker J, Veltri EP, et al. Clinical interaction between pacemakers and automatic implantable cardioverter-defibrillators. *J Am Coll Cardiol* 1990;16:666.

Cappato R. Secondary prevention of sudden death: the Dutch study, the Antiarrhythmics Versus Implantable Defibrillator Trial, the Cardiac Arrest Study Hamburg, and the Canadian Implantable Defibrillator Study. *Am J Cardiol* 1999;83:68D.

Dreifus LS, Fisch C, Griffin JC, et al. Guidelines for implantation of cardiac pacemakers and antiarrhythmia devices: a report of the American College of Cardiology/American Heart Association Task Force on assessment of diagnostic and therapeutic cardiovascular procedures (Committee on pacemaker implantation). *Circulation* 1991;84:455, and *J Am Coll Cardiol* 1991;18:1.

Embil JM, Geddes JS, Foster D, Sandeman J. Return to arc welding following defibrillator implantation. *Pacing Clin Electrophysiol* 1993;16:2313.

Exner D, Yee R, Jones DL, et al. Combination biphasic waveform plus sequential pulse defibrillation improves defibrillation efficacy of a nonthoracotomy lead system. *J Am Coll Cardiol* 1994;23:317.

Fisher JD, Kim SG, Waspe LE, Matos JA. Mechanisms for the success and failure of pacing for termination of ventricular tachycardia: clinical and hypothetical considerations (Part II). *Pacing Clin Electrophysiol* 1983;6:1094.

Furman S. Implantable cardioverter defibrillator infection (Part I). *Pacing Clin Electrophysiol* 1990;13: 1351.

Geelen P, Lorga A, Chauvin M, Wellens F, Brugada P. The value of DDD pacing in patients with an implantable cardioverter defibrillator (Part II). *Pacing Clin Electrophysiol* 1997;20:177.

Higgins S, Williams S, Pak J, Meyer D. Indications for implantation of a dual-chamber pacemaker combined with an implantable cardioverter-defibrillator. *Am J Cardiol* 1998;81:1360.

Heisel A, Jung J. The atrial defibrillator: a stand-alone device or part of a combined dual-chamber system? *Am J Cardiol* 1999;83:218D.

Jung W, Manz M, Pfeiffer D, et al. Effects of antiarrhythmic drugs on epicardial defibrillation energy requirements and the rate of defibrillator discharges (Part II). *Pacing Clin Electrophysiol* 1993;16:198.

KenKnight B, Jones B, Thomas A, Lang D. Technological advances in implantable cardioverter-defibrillators before the year 2000 and beyond. *Am J Cardiol* 1996;78:108.

Keren R, Aaron SP, Veltri EP. Anxiety and depression in patients with life-threatening ventricular arrhythmias: impact of the ICD. *Pacing Clin Electrophysiol* 1991;14:181.

Kron J, Silka MJ, Ohm O-J, et al. Preliminary experience with nonthoracotomy implantable cardioverter defibrillators in young patients. *Pacing Clin Electrophysiol* 1994;17:26.

Lehmann MH, Saksena S, for the NASPE Policy Conference Committee. Implantable cardioverter defibrillators in cardiovascular practice: report of the policy conference of the North American Society of Pacing and Electrophysiology (NASPE) Policy Conference Committee. *Pacing Clin Electrophysiol* 1991;14:969.

Leitch JW, Gillis AM, Wyse G, et al. Reduction in defibrillator shock with an implantable device combining antitachycardia pacing and shock therapy. *J Am Coll Cardiol* 1991;18:145.

Mirowski M, Reid PR, Mower MM, et al. Clinical performance of the implantable cardioverter-defibrillator (Part II). *Pacing Clin Electrophysiol* 1984;7:1345.

Morris M, KenKnight B, Warren J, Lang D. A preview of implantable cardioverter defibrillator systems in the next millennium: an integrative cardiac rhythm management approach. *Am J Cardiol* 1999; 83:48D.

Moss A, Zareba W. Implantable defibrillators for prevention of sudden cardiac death. In: Califf R, Isner J, Prsytowsky E, et al., eds. *Textbook of cardiovascular medicine*. Philadelphia: Lippincott–Raven, 1998.

Moss AJ, ed. Automatic implantable cardioverter defibrillator (Part I). *Prog Cardiovasc Dis* 1993;36:85.

Moss AJ, ed. Automatic implantable cardioverter defibrillator (Part II). *Prog Cardiovasc Dis* 1993;36:179.

Myerburg R, Castellanos A. A comparison of antiarrhythmic-drug therapy with implantable defibrillators in patients resuscitated from near-fatal ventricular arrhythmias. *N Engl J Med* 1997;337:1576.

Nair M, Saoudi N, Kroiss D, Letac B. Automatic arrhythmia identification using analysis of the atrioventricular association. *Circulation* 1997;95:967.

Saxon L, Boehmer J, Hummel J, et al. Biventricular pacing in patients with congestive heart failure: two prospective randomized trials. *Am J Cardiol* 1999;83:120D.

Shahian DM, Williamson WA, Martin D, Venditti FJ Jr. Infection of implantable cardioverter defibrillator systems: a preventable complication? *Pacing Clin Electrophysiol* 1993;16:1956.

Strickberger SA, Cantillon CO, Friedman PL. Should sudden death survivors resume driving? Analysis of state laws and physician practices. *Pacing Clin Electrophysiol* 1991;14:720(abst).

Tavernier R, Jordaens L. The clinical experience with the Metrix automatic implantable atrial defibrillator. *J Am Coll Cardiol* 1998;195A(abst).

Teplitz L, Egenes KJ, Brask L. Life after sudden death: the development of a support group for automatic implantable cardioverter-defibrillator patients. *J Cardiovasc Nurs* 1990;4:20.

Thakur RK, Souza JJ, Troup PJ, et al. Pericardial effusion increases defibrillation energy requirement. *Pacing Clin Electrophysiol* 1993;16:1227.

Trappe H, Achtelik M, Pfitzner P, Voigt B, Weismuller P. Single-chamber versus dual-chamber implantable cardioverter defibrillators: indications and clinical results. *Am J Cardiol* 1999;83:8D.

Winkle RA, Mead RH, Ruder MA, et al. Improved low energy defibrillation efficacy with the use of a biphasic truncated exponential waveform. *Am Heart J* 1989;117:122.

Yamanouchi Y, Brewer J, Mowrey K, Donohoo A, Wilkoff B, Tchou P. Optimal small-capacitor biphasic waveform for external defibrillation. *Circulation* 1998;98:2487.

9

Pacemaker Implantation

PERMANENT PACEMAKER IMPLANTATION

Permanent Transvenous Pacing

Transvenous pacing in the VVI mode has become the standard by which other pacing methods are measured. Tined leads that have soft barbs at the electrode end have become widely used because of their low rate of dislodgment (see Fig. 2-3). Before the development of grasping leads, a lead dislodgment rate of 10% to 30% was not unusual and was a major objection to the use of transvenous rather than transthoracic pacing.

Most frequently, to place a lead for permanent pacing, the cephalic vein is located and cannulated in the deltopectoral groove with the patient under local anesthesia (Fig. 9-1). Less commonly, the internal or external jugular vein is used. Under fluoroscopic imaging, the electrode can be guided into the apex of the right ventricle. Satisfactory thresholds are documented by measurement with a pacing system analyzer rather than with a temporary pacemaker. The minimum voltage necessary to capture the ventricle is determined; usually, it is less than 1 V (and preferably less than 0.5 V) when the pulse width is set between 0.5 and 0.8 msec. The electric resistance or impedance in ohms can be calculated. (Most pacing system analyzers will do this automatically.) This value reflects the resistance of the lead and the electrode–myocardial interface (polarization resistance). The amplitude of the patient's intrinsically generated QRS pattern then is measured. To be recognized by the pacemaker for proper ventricular inhibition function, the amplitude must be of sufficient size. Usually, no problems are encountered in finding a value exceeding 4 mV that allows sensing with a reasonable safety margin (Table 3-1). The leads are attached to the pulse generator, and a pocket is fashioned by separating the pectoral muscle fascia from the overlying subcutaneous tissue. The subcutaneous tissue and skin are closed in layers. After a short course of prophylactic antibiotics, the patient can be discharged from the hospital and has follow-up in a pacemaker clinic.

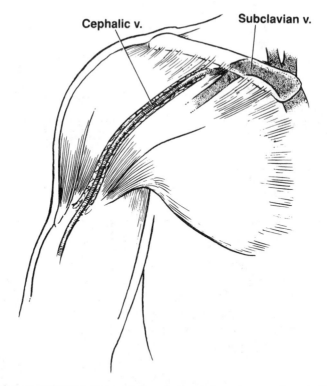

FIG. 9-1. Deltopectoral groove. The cephalic vein travels from the arm, through the deltopectoral groove, and joins the subclavian vein. It is located easily in most patients.

Atrial pacing leads are being implanted with increasing frequency. This kind of lead almost always is implanted simultaneously with a ventricular lead but positioned in the atrial appendage. When attached to a dual-chamber pacemaker, sequential atrial and ventricular contraction can be electrically timed to stimulate normal physiology. (The rationale for this approach is discussed in Chapter 6.) If the atrial J lead is used, the lead is advanced with the stylet in place to the lower right atrium near the tricuspid valve. The stylet should be withdrawn and the tip positioned anteriorly as the lead assumes its J shape. The lead then can be pulled back slightly to engage the right atrial appendage. The tip should be stable in the right atrial appendage with gentle rotational movement of the lead and with deep breaths by the patient. With a deep breath, the angle of the J should not open to more than 90 degrees. Lateral fluoroscopy should show the tip to be in an anterior position.

With a pulse width of 0.5 to 0.8 msec, the voltage threshold should be lower than 1.5 V, preferably below 1.0 V. The sensed P wave should be greater than 1.5 mV (see Table 3-1).

The following methods may be used to document atrial capture:

1. Observance of a P wave on the surface electrocardiogram (ECG) following the pacemaker spike. Sometimes this is difficult to see, especially if the atrial lead is unipolar, with a large spike distorting the baseline. If an electrophysiologic study is being done, an intraatrial lead can be used to demonstrate a large P wave.

2. The presence of a QRS complex occurring consistently after each atrial spike, with a short delay between the spike and the QRS complex. Obviously, this method is of no use in patients with AV heart block.

3. Documentation of atrial contraction by fluoroscopy. The atrium may be seen to contract with lateral movement of the atrial lead during atrial contraction.

The order of positioning the atrial and ventricular leads is partly personal preference. If the ventricular lead is placed first, it is available for emergency use during the procedure. The threshold and sensing values of the first-placed lead should be rechecked after the second lead is stabilized to ensure that no minor dislodgment has occurred.

A new type of introducer with a peel-away sheath often is used for permanent transvenous lead placement. A subclavian venous puncture is performed, a guidewire is passed into the subclavian vein, and a dilator and sheath are advanced over the guidewire into the vein. The guidewire and dilator then are removed, and the sheath is left in the vein for passage of the pacing lead. This technique is used routinely by cardiologists for access to a large vein or artery and is referred to as the *Seldinger technique*. The lead can be advanced to the heart through the sheath, and sometimes both atrial and ventricular leads are placed through a single sheath. The sheath then can be split apart and discarded to allow connection of the lead to the generator (Fig. 9-2).

The subclavian technique may be technically easier if the cephalic vein is difficult to localize. On the other hand, it carries the potential disadvantages of pneumothorax, possibly with tension pneumothorax, air embolism, nerve injury, hemopneumothorax, and puncture of the lymphatic vessels. It is possible that fewer wire fractures may occur with a cephalic vein cutdown because the angle of this pacemaker lead from the generator to the vessel may be gentler.

A potential problem with the subclavian technique is the risk of "crush" injury. If the pacemaker lead is placed too medially, it will be secured between the first rib and clavicle too tightly, which can lead to lead fracture. The lead fracture is probably not due to true crushing, but to firm fixation of the lead in that area with the more distal part of the lead being mobile, with chronic motion leading to lead fracture. The lead must not be placed too medially.

Permanent Transthoracic Pacing

If the need for permanent pacing is identified when cardiac surgery is performed, direct attachment of the pacing leads to the heart's myocardium is a

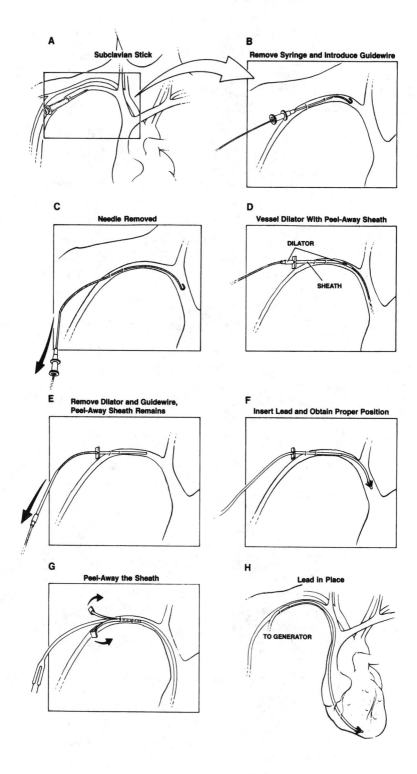

straightforward matter. The appropriate electrode may be sutured to the heart; more commonly, the screw-in lead (see Fig. 2-6) is attached to the "bare area" of the right ventricle, an area on the diaphragmatic surface of the ventricle that is invariably free of the fat that otherwise covers most of the chamber. Occasionally, the thresholds from this area are not satisfactory, and placement of electrodes in other locations, usually on the left ventricle, is accomplished. Pacing thresholds are determined in the same manner as for transvenous pacing. The pacing leads are placed under the sternum, and a pacemaker pocket is developed in the upper abdominal quadrant, usually on the left, above the rectus fascia. Occasionally, permanent pacing wires, attached at the time of open heart surgery, are left above the rectus fascia, unattached to a pulse generator unit. These wires can be located later under local anesthesia, and permanent pacing can be initiated simply by connecting them to a pulse generator unit.

Myocardial lead placement is always the best option when satisfactory placement of a transvenous lead is not possible because of chamber dilation, the presence of a prosthetic tricuspid valve, or lack of suitable venous access; nor is it the best option in growing children. Two approaches for myocardial lead insertion generally are used when the primary objective is to establish myocardial pacing. By far the most common approach used is transxiphoid. Under a local or light general anesthesia, the xiphoid process is exposed by a short, midline, lower sternal incision. Its excision facilitates exposure of the pericardial surface that is opened, allowing the leads to be attached directly to the bare area of the right ventricle. The pacemaker then is placed in a pocket developed in the left upper abdominal quadrant above the rectus fascia. Occasionally, an anterior left thoracotomy incision, exposing the left ventricle between the fifth and sixth interspace, is indicated. Electrodes are then attached to the left ventricular myocardium and tunneled to the abdominal wall, where they can be attached to a pulse generator (Fig. 9-3).

The implanter should be aware of the fact that if the seal on the sterilized pacemaker leads is broken, most manufacturers will assume that he or she has bought the device even if it is not placed in the patient. The implanter may want to contact the company in this situation to minimize consternation.

FIG. 9-2. Subclavian stick technique with peel-away sheath. A needle is placed into the subclavian vein (see text for proper positioning), and a guidewire is advanced through the needle into the subclavian vein and superior vena cava. The needle is removed, and a dilator with a peel-away sheath around it is advanced through the skin into the vein. The guidewire and dilator then are removed, leaving the peel-away sheath in place. A lead or leads can be advanced through the sheath and placed in the proper position. The advantage of the peel-away sheath is that it can be removed, peeled in half, and discarded. The pacemaker lead then is attached to the generator subcutaneously and the skin is closed. This technique can be used anytime, although we generally use it when there is difficulty locating a proper cephalic vein. Also, for dual-chamber pacemakers, this approach allows two leads to be placed with relative ease (often the cephalic vein is of adequate size for only one lead).

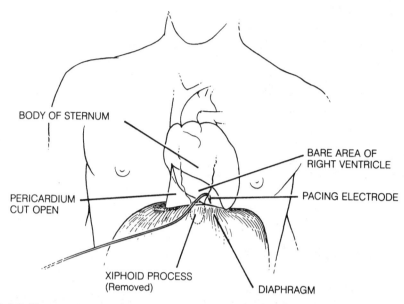

BODY OF STERNUM

BARE AREA OF
RIGHT VENTRICLE

PERICARDIUM
CUT OPEN

PACING ELECTRODE

XIPHOID PROCESS
(Removed)

DIAPHRAGM

FIG. 9-3. The transxiphoid approach is used to place epicardial pacemaker leads. The xiphoid process itself is removed, exposing the bare area of the right ventricle. The epicardial screw-in leads can be placed in this area, and the generator itself is placed subcutaneously in the abdomen.

Lead and Generator Connection

The attachment of the electrode to the generator is an important step in pacemaker implantation. A typical connection is shown in Figure 9-4. The exposed metal portion of the connector is inserted into the pulse generator. The insertion must be complete, and the metal wire and insulating material should fit snugly into the socket. This tight fit avoids fluid intrusion into the connection. A metal set screw is screwed down to complete the connection. Finally, an insulating plastic plug is placed over the metal set screw to prevent fluid intrusion that could lead to a short circuit in the system or corrosion of the connection. Modifications of this type of attachment are present in various pacemaker models. As noted in Chapter 10, improper connection of the electrode to the pulse generator, or problems occurring at this connection, can lead to a variety of pacemaker malfunctions.

The system shown in Figure 9-4 is not commonly used, but it shows the principle that the set screw must firmly connect the exposed metal wire to the pacemaker generator, and then the set screw must be insulated. Commonly, devices now have built-in insulation with a special screwdriver that can turn the screw through the insulation. Also commonly, a "torque wrench" is used so that the set screw cannot be overtightened, leading to damage. At least one manufacturer has an automatic locking system.

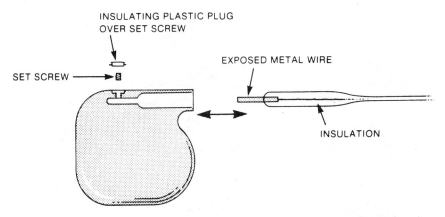

FIG. 9-4. This figure is schematic; for instance, the international connecting lead is not shown and usually the insulating plug is not mobile. The concept, however, remains the same. Material is placed permanently over the set screw, which then is tightened with a specially designed screwdriver through the insulating material.

Perioperative Care

Care needs after transvenous placement of a pacemaker are minimal. Antibiotics are given routinely through the perioperative phase, and constant monitoring of the heart rhythm is desirable to detect any failure to capture the heart or failure of the pacemaker sensing functions. Not infrequently, intrinsic arrhythmias must be treated. A postoperative chest radiograph documents the position of the pacing lead and can be used for comparison if pacemaker lead migration is suspected in the future. Figure 9-5 demonstrates typical positioning of an atrial J lead in the right atrial appendage and of a right ventricular lead.

Complications

As with all surgical procedures, complications are possible and should be reviewed with the patient before consent for the procedure is done. Pacing complications relating to electric pacing malfunctions are discussed in Chapter 10. The surgical possibilities of hemorrhage and infection occur rarely. Hemorrhage as a major complication is more prevalent with the transxiphoid or thoracotomy approach than with a transvenous approach. Arrhythmias, especially ventricular tachycardia, occur frequently during seating of the lead, but these are rarely a problem of any consequence.

It is often observed that once ventricular pacing is initiated, the heart becomes pacemaker dependent for a period. Therefore, after electrical capture is begun, repositioning of the lead should be done with caution.

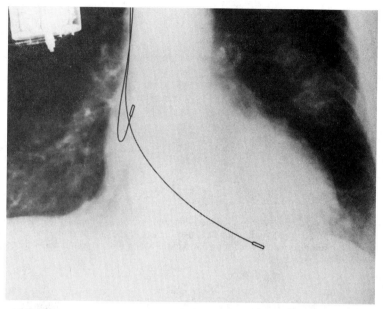

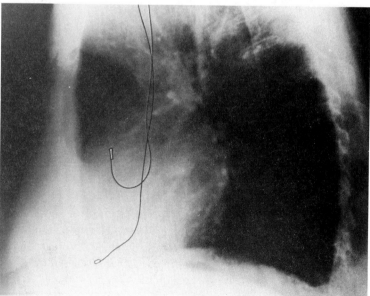

FIG. 9-5. Position of atrial and ventricular leads on the chest radiograph. The atrial J lead is positioned in the right atrial appendage and travels anteriorly and slightly medially. The ventricular lead is in the right ventricular apex. A ventricular lead inadvertently placed in the coronary sinus rather than the right ventricular apex could appear to be in good position on the posterior–anterior view on a chest radiograph or fluoroscopy but on the lateral view would be posterior rather than anterior.

Although infection is uncommon, removal of the pulse generator and lead often is necessary to eradicate infection when it does occur. Pacemaker erosion may occur in the absence of infection.

Generator Change

With today's long-lived pacemaker generators, it is common for the patient to die with the original pacemaker still functioning. Battery depletion or other problems may require the pulse generator to be removed. The most frequent indication for removal is battery depletion (particularly with the greater use of dual-chamber pacemakers, but some rate-responsive pacemakers also tend to deplete their energy source more quickly). Usually, there has been an indicator during telephone follow-up (e.g., a drop in magnet rate, pulse width change, or mode change) that the battery is near end of life.

When the generator is changed, it is prudent to make a decision as to whether the current pacing mode is still appropriate. At the same time, the pacing lead should be critically analyzed and the pacemaker generator pocket evaluated. It is possible that a DDD pacemaker may best be changed to a VVI or a VVIR if the patient has developed chronic atrial fibrillation, for instance. The atrial lead then could be capped or removed.

The compatibility of the "hardware" needs to be considered. The lead, pin, and connector compatibility between the old lead system and the new generator lead may influence the decision as to which pulse generator to select. An international standard is being developed to produce leads, pins, and connectors that should simplify this decision process.

The electric characteristics of the lead itself should be evaluated, and the operator should be sure to what extent the patient is pacemaker dependent (i.e., the patient may need temporary pacing immediately once the generator is disconnected). If the pulse generator has become battery exhausted long before its predicted life span, a lead problem (e.g., a lead insulator fault that has led to very low impedance and high energy drain from the battery) should be suspected. The chronically implanted lead is tested in a manner identical to that of a new lead with an analyzer system to measure voltage threshold, current threshold, calculated resistance of the lead, and voltage of the sensed electrograms.

Modern leads appear to have better "chronic thresholds" than do leads of older design; however, every lead should be evaluated on its own merits. Also, it should be determined that the lead in place is not one that has been recalled by the manufacturer due to a higher-than-expected incidence of problems.

If the lead threshold is greater than 2.5 V, consideration should be given to a lead replacement to allow an adequate safety margin of pacemaker output and also to provide the potential for longer life of the pulse generator. Although several manufacturers make high-output generators to afford function to patients with high chronic thresholds, their use is not as desirable as replacement of the lead to achieve a low threshold.

Perhaps the least common lead problem is having good chronic thresholds but poorly sensed electrograms. Sometimes satisfactory function may be obtained from such a lead by using it as a unipolar lead rather than a bipolar lead with appropriate choice of pacemakers or pacemaker program configuration in the unipolar mode. The unipolar configuration results in a longer antenna for sensing electrograms but may be more susceptible, therefore, to extraneous signals.

Three things may be done with a lead that has been replaced:

1. It may be removed. This is often possible with screw-in leads and usually is impossible with chronic leads of the tine variety. If the lead is infected, extra effort is appropriate in attempting to remove the lead. Anecdotal reports of successful removal of chronically stuck leads by up to a few days of traction with 1 to 2 pounds of weight have been reported; however, brute force to remove the lead is dangerous because it may result in myocardial tricuspid valve damage, and such force is not appropriate.
2. Capping the lead and replacing the pulse generator pocket is a common way of dealing with a replaced lead. The cap prevents extraneous electric currents from entering the unshielded wire. The disadvantage of the capping option is that it increases the bulk in the pulse-generator pocket.
3. Often the lead can be cut short and the exposed wire trimmed so that the insulation can be brought over the exposed wire and sealed by medical silicone glue. Although this does not remove the wire from the superior vena cava and heart, it eliminates the bulk in the pulse-generator pocket. This approach is usually well tolerated.

The pulse-generator pocket itself should be evaluated at every replacement operation. It is often advantageous to incise the capsule at the inferior margin of the pulse generator pocket to allow the new generator to be placed without undue skin tension at the suture line. Pulse generators that have migrated into the axilla or the breast should be relocated to a more suitable position and the generator itself then sutured to the chest wall.

Care of the patient for generator lead pocket revision is identical to that of a patient with a fresh implant. The pacemaker follow-up facility should be notified of the operation and of any and all changes made in hardware or software programming at the time of the cardiac pacemaker revision.

TEMPORARY PACEMAKER PLACEMENT

Emergency Pacing

Although the judicious use of cardiac pacing can be lifesaving and often is needed urgently, its effectiveness in the setting of cardiac resuscitation is separate from its usual implementation. True emergency pacing, as used in this discussion, does not refer to situations in which it is feared that failure to initiate pacing immediately will result in catastrophic hemodynamic deterioration, but rather to those desperate situations in which catastrophic hemodynamic deterioration has already occurred and prolonged cardiac standstill is recognized. Of course, standard cardiopulmonary resuscitation methods with establishment of airway and chest compression are indicated.

The failure of chronotropic drug therapy (e.g., atropine and isoproterenol) to support the circulation is an ominous sign. The use of electrical pacing may be lifesaving in this situation, and transthoracic pacing is the most direct method. A common system is one in which a single wire is introduced by a percutaneous puncture into the ventricular chamber, with an approach nearly identical to that used for pericardiocentesis.

The needle is withdrawn, leaving the pacing wire in contact with the myocardium. A second subcutaneous metal needle serves as the anode terminal to complete the pacing circuit. (Bipolar transthoracic pacing wires are also available.) Assuming the electrode is properly placed, pacing can be initiated within 1 minute; however, patients in cardiac standstill who have a primary injury other than interruption of a cardiac conduction system, such as massive myocardial infarction with cardiogenic shock, acidosis, or terminal arrhythmias of other origin, may not benefit from transthoracic pacing. Possible complications of this approach include pneumothorax, hemothorax, coronary artery laceration, and cardiac tamponade; it is a route to be used only in desperate situations. Nevertheless, the equipment and technical facility to initiate transthoracic pacing should be part of every cardiac care unit's emergency capability.

Other routes for establishing emergency pacing are the subclavian and internal jugular veins. Often, a pacing lead can be passed blindly from these central veins to the right ventricular apex. If the patient has an intrinsic rhythm, the V lead of the ECG can be attached to the pacing lead to help locate the position of the electrode. A giant P wave indicates that the pacing tip is in the right atrium, and a giant QRS complex indicates that it is in the right ventricle. Whenever conditions permit, however, use of fluoroscopy is always preferable. The transcutaneous pacemaker (described in Chapter 5) offers an excellent alternative to the approach just described and is becoming the most commonly used method of emergency pacing (see Figs. 5-5 and 5-6).

Temporary Transvenous Pacing

For temporary pacing under less emergent circumstances, the route of access can be through a venous cutdown (usually an antecubital vein) or by the percutaneous Seldinger venipuncture technique into the subclavian, femoral, or jugular vein. Percutaneous puncture of the femoral vein is perhaps the safest and easiest route. The femoral vein is in constant relationship to the femoral artery at the inguinal canal because it is medial to the femoral artery pulsation as it crosses under the inguinal ligament (see Fig. 9-6). Confirmation of venous puncture by the color and pressure of the blood return and, under fluoroscopy, by the

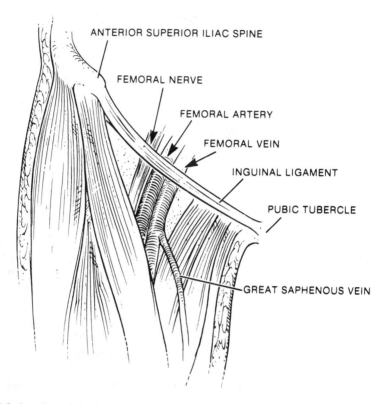

ANTERIOR SUPERIOR ILIAC SPINE

FEMORAL NERVE

FEMORAL ARTERY

FEMORAL VEIN

INGUINAL LIGAMENT

PUBIC TUBERCLE

GREAT SAPHENOUS VEIN

FIG. 9-6. Location of the femoral vein. The femoral vein usually can be entered easily just medial to the femoral artery pulse in the femoral crease.

characteristic course of the catheter to the right of the vertebral column assures that inadvertent arterial puncture has not occurred.

Excellent temporary vascular access also is achieved through the subclavian vein (Fig. 9-7). The subclavian vein has become a standard route of venous access because the anterior scalene muscle separates the subclavian artery posteriorly from the subclavian vein anteriorly at the base of the neck. Selective venous puncture can be achieved reliably by guiding the exploring needle behind the clavicle and aiming toward the suprasternal notch. It is wise to avoid subclavian puncture in patients who have undergone anticoagulation or who have coagulation defects, who are restless, or who could not tolerate a pneumothorax. Technically, this procedure may be difficult if the clavicle has been previously fractured, if the patient has severe vasospasm, or if the patient is hypovolemic. The Trendelenburg position enlarges the vein and enhances the chance of successful venous puncture. At the same time, the Trendelenburg position reduces the chance of air embolism. If a chest tube is in place for another reason, it is

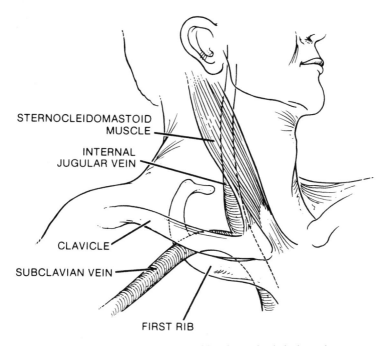

FIG. 9-7. Location of the internal jugular and subclavian veins.

wise to perform the subclavian puncture on the same side as the chest tube. The chest tube then treats, in advance, the most common complications (pneumothorax and hemothorax) of the procedure. Inexperience and multiple attempts at subclavian venous puncture are additive in producing complications.

The internal jugular vein also can be used successfully for transvenous access for a pacing catheter. Knowledge of the anatomy of the jugular vein at the base of the neck is essential to the successful use of this route. By guiding a needle deep into the sternocleidomastoid muscle and between the sternal and clavicular heads of the sternocleidomastoid muscle, the vein usually can be located easily (see Fig. 9-7). Steep Trendelenburg position facilitates successful puncture of the vein. Complications include carotid artery puncture, hemothorax, or pneumothorax. Left-sided venous puncture has the additional theoretic hazard of possible injury to the thoracic duct at its juncture with the left jugular vein.

An antecubital cutdown is a time-tested and reliable way to achieve temporary transvenous pacing (Fig. 9-8). The cephalic, basilic, and median cubital veins are usually located with ease in the subcutaneous tissue of the antecubital space. The basilic vein offers the most direct route into the subclavian vein and is the preferable arm vein, but this route may be less stable, because of arm movement, than those already mentioned.

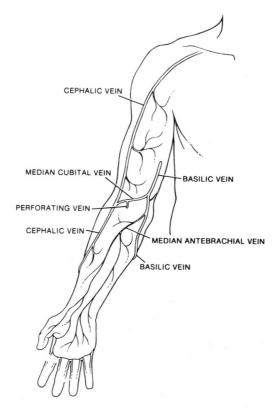

FIG. 9-8. Arm veins. The basilic vein provides the most direct route into the subclavian vein from the arm.

Either the standard bipolar temporary transvenous lead or the newer balloon-guided electrode can be introduced once a venous conduit is secured. Placement of a pacing lead should be guided and checked by fluoroscopic imaging.

Temporary Pacing after Cardiac Surgery

Often after cardiac surgery, temporary pacing wires are fixed directly to the epicardium or myocardium or both. These wires generally are insulated in containers when not used but are readily available if perioperative pacing becomes desirable. Three patterns of wire placement are common. The simplest is a single myocardial wire (unipolar lead) that must be used with a ground wire, using a small-gauge wire stitch or metal needle in the adjacent subcutaneous tissue. Alternatively, two myocardial leads, usually attached to the anterior right ventricle, may be used. This allows placement of a bipolar pacing lead. Either wire can be used as the anode (+) or cathode (−); if one wire fails, the system can be converted to a unipolar lead system. Finally, two pairs of temporary pacing wires can be used for atrioventricular sequential pacing. In this system, a bipolar atrial and bipolar ventricular pair of wires are placed so that maximum cardiac output can be achieved by use with the atrioventricular sequential (DVI) temporary pulse generator.

Recording from an atrial lead, when available, can be quite helpful in the diagnosis of tachycardias. By attaching an atrial lead to the V lead terminal of a standard electrocardiograph, the large atrial waves can be seen easily and can be used to distinguish among various types of supraventricular arrhythmias. These temporary leads are removed simply by pulling them out. Hemorrhage is a rare problem.

REFERENCES

Astridge PS, Kaye GC, Whitworth S, et al. The response of implanted dual chamber pacemakers to 50 Hz extravenous electrical interferences. *Pacing Clin Electrophysiol* 1993;16:1966.

Camunas J, Mehta D, Ip J, et al. Total pectoral implantation: a new technique for implantation of transvenous defibrillator lead systems and implantable cardioverter defibrillator (Part I). *Pacing Clin Electrophysiol* 1993;16:1380.

Costa A, Kirkorian G, Cucherat M, Delahaye F, et al. Antibiotic prophylaxis for permanent pacemaker implantation. *Circulation* 1998;97:1796.

Da Costa A, Lelievre H, Kirkorian G. Role of the preaxillary flora in pacemaker infections. *Circulation* 1998;97:1791.

Epstein M, Walsh E, Saul J, Triedman J, Mayer J, Gamble W. Long-term performance of bipolar epicardial atrial pacing using an active fixation bipolar endocardial lead (Part II). *Pacing Clin Electrophysiol* 1998;21:1098.

Faust M, Fraser, Schurig L, et al. Educational guidelines for the clinically associated professional in cardiac pacing and electrophysiology (Part I). *Pacing Clin Electrophysiol* 1990;13:1448.

Frumin H, Goodman GR, Pleatman M. ICD implantation via thoracoscopy without the need for sternotomy or thoracotomy. *Pacing Clin Electrophysiol* 1993;16:257.

Fyke FE III. Infraclavicular lead failure: tarnish on a golden route (Part I). *Pacing Clin Electrophysiol* 1993;16:373.

Gold M. Optimization of ventricular pacing: where should we implant the leads? *J Am Coll Cardiol* 1999; 33:324.

Greene TO, Portnow AS, Huang SKS. Acute pericarditis resulting from an endocardial active fixation screw-in atrial lead. *Pacing Clin Electrophysiol* 1994;17:21.

Hayes DL, Naccarelli GV, Furman S, Parsonnet V. Report of the NASPE policy conference: training requirements for permanent pacemaker selection, implantation, and follow-up. *Pacing Clin Electrophysiol* 1994;17:6.

Jacobs DM, Fink AS, Miller RP, et al. Anatomical and morphological evaluation of pacemaker lead compression (Part I). *Pacing Clin Electrophysiol* 1993;16:434.

Jamidar H, Goli V, Reynolds DW. The right atrial free wall: an alternative pacing site (Part I). *Pacing Clin Electrophysiol* 1993;16:959.

Josephson M, Maloney J, Barold S, et al. Task Force 6: training in specialized electrophysiology, cardiac pacing and arrhythmia management. *J Am Coll Cardiol* 1995;25:23.

Magney JE, Staplin DH, Flynn DM, Hunter DW. A new approach to percutaneous subclavian venipuncture to avoid lead fracture or central venous catheter occlusion. *Pacing Clin Electrophysiol* 1993;16: 2133.

Manolis A, Chiladakis J, Vassilikos V, Maounis T, Cokkinos D. Pectoral cardioverter defibrillators: comparison of prepectoral and submuscular implantation techniques. *Pacing Clin Electrophysiol* 1999;22:469.

Ohm O-J, Breivik K, Hammer EA, Hoff PI. Intraoperative electrical measurements during pacemaker implantation. *Clin Prog Pacing Electrophysiol* 1984;2:1.

O'Sullivan JJ, Jameson S, Gold RG, Wren C. Endocardial pacemakers in children: lead length and allowance for growth. *Pacing Clin Electrophysiol* 1993;16:267.

Schwaab B, Frohlig G, Alexander C, et al. Influence of right ventricular stimulation site on left ventricular function in atrial synchronous ventricular pacing. *J Am Coll Cardiol* 1999;33:317.

van Gelder BM, Bracke FALE, ElGamel MIH. Adapter failure as a cause of pacemaker malfunction. *Pacing Clin Electrophysiol* 1993;16:1961.

Victor F, Leclercq C, Mabo P, et al. Optimal right ventricular pacing site in chronically implanted patients. *J Am Coll Cardiol* 1999;33:311.

Ward DE, Jones S, Shinebourne EA. Long-term transvenous pacing in children weighing ten kilograms or less. *Int J Cardiol* 1987;15:112.

Zoll PM. Resuscitation of the heart in ventricular standstill by external electric stimulation. *N Engl J Med* 1952;247:768.

10

Follow-up of the Patient Who Has Received a Pacemaker

INITIAL PACEMAKER CLINIC FOLLOW-UP VISIT

An organized system of follow-up is important for all pacemaker patients and is best facilitated through the patient's membership in a formal pacemaker follow-up clinic. The first formal clinic follow-up visit is usually scheduled at approximately 2 to 3 months after implantation to allow for completion of the lead-tissue maturation process, which may affect sensing and capture thresholds and reprogramming, to account for the threshold change, and still provide a safety margin along with improved battery life. The patient generally will have additional questions at this time, and the pocket can be evaluated for appropriate healing. The initial evaluation begins with a limited history and physical examination.

History and Physical

The history should focus on symptoms related to impaired cardiac output that may reflect potential pacemaker malfunction. These include palpitations, dizziness, presyncope/syncope, or any symptom that may resemble those experienced preimplantation. The possibility of pacemaker syndrome always should be considered a potention cause for recurrent or new symptoms. Complaints related to potential pacemaker infection also should be explored, including fever, chills, recurrent respiratory illness, or the report of swelling, drainage, or tenderness in the region of the pocket. Table 10-1 lists some symptoms that should lead to the suspicion of potential problems. Fortunately, these problems are quite rare.

The examination consists of measuring vital signs and inspecting the pocket area. Attention should be paid to the presence of localized tenderness, swelling, or redness. The patient may complain of symptoms related to progression of their underlying cardiac disease so that the follow-up visit presents an opportunity for reevaluation of the patient's general cardiac status.

143

TABLE 10–1. *Symptoms that may alert the clinician to pacemaker problems*

Patient symptoms	Consider
I have a constant hiccup	Diaphragmatic pacing
My shoulder jumps	Pectoral muscle pacing
My pacemaker is sore	Pacemaker pocket infection
I am sick	Pacemaker lead infection
My arm hurts	Brachial plexus irritation
My heart is racing	Pacemaker-mediated tachycardia or other tachycardias unrelated to the pacemaker
I am dizzy	Loss of capture or inappropriate bradycardia
My pacemaker has moved (and is in my armpit, lower chest, etc.)	Pacemaker migration

Electrocardiogram

An electrocardiographic tracing should be obtained and can be done using a 12-lead electrocardiograph, but a single-lead rhythm strip demonstrating visible P waves is usually adequate because additional recordings may be necessary during the visit. The recording will disclose whether the patient is presently being paced and in what manner. If not, the underlying rhythm and the PR interval can be established.

Figure 10-1 depicts a unipolar spike causing distortion of the baseline, which could be mistaken for true capture. Bipolar spikes tend to be smaller than unipolar spikes (because the electricity is traveling the shorter distance through the body) and may be harder to identify. If the patient is in a clinic, a look at various leads of the electrocardiogram (ECG) may clarify the presence or absence of capture. In the case of confusing rhythm strips received over the telephone, clarifica-

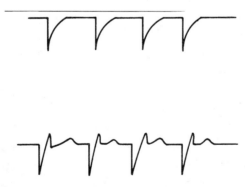

FIG. 10-1. Unipolar pacemaker rhythm strip. **Top:** A unipolar pacemaker with a large pacemaker spike and distorted baseline due to after-potential. There is no capture of the heart during this time. The distorted baseline can be mistaken for a QRS complex. **Bottom:** A rhythm strip in the same patient with repositioning of the lead and capture of the patient's heart. Note the appearance of a T wave, which is often helpful in identifying true capture in this situation.

tion may be possible by placing a chest-wall transmitter on various parts of the body to change the rhythm strip configuration or by using fingertip electrodes.

Fusion and pseudofusion beats are shown in Figure 10-2. A fusion beat is a QRS complex that has been formed by depolarization of the myocardium, initiated by both the pacemaker spike and the patient's intrinsic beat. A pseudofusion beat is a QRS complex that is formed by a depolarization of the myocardium initiated by a patient's intrinsic heartbeat completely; however, a pacemaker spike is present, distorting the QRS complex. These can be normal occurrences in pacemaker patients.

Magnet Rate

To obtain the magnet rate, a standard magnet is applied over the pocket area for a brief period. The presence of the magnetic field causes a switch to temporarily convert the pacemaker into the VOO (asynchronous pacing) or DOO mode in the case of a DDD device. The rate at which the pacemaker fires during the magnet application depends on the model of the pacemaker. Some models fire at a slower rate than the programmed rate, whereas others fire at the same or at a faster rate. A common question raised by clinicians concerns the safety of using the magnet mode because, theoretically, a pacing spike occurring on the T wave could induce ventricular arrhythmias. This is rarely a practical problem, however, and the common use of magnet mode during transtelephonic evaluations has been shown to be quite safe.

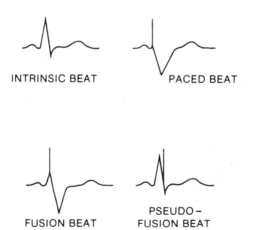

FIG. 10-2. Fusion and pseudofusion beats. Intrinsic beats and paced beats are shown (**top**). A fusion beat is a combination of the patient's intrinsic beat and a paced beat. A pseudofusion beat is a QRS complex caused by an intrinsic beat that is distorted by the patient's spike, which does not obviously depolarize the myocardium. These findings are normal and do not represent pacemaker malfunction.

Pacemaker Interrogation

The device then should be interrogated to establish the programmed parameters. The interrogation also should include a list of variables collectively referred to as *measured data*, which include lead information (atrial or ventricular) such as pulse amplitude (volts), current, and impedance. Both the programmed parameters and measured data should be printed, filed in the patient's chart, and labeled to distinguish this information from a printed summary generated at the end of the visit to document any reprogrammed parameters.

Establishing the Underlying Rhythm

The next step is to establish the patient's underlying rhythm and to determine whether the individual is pacemaker dependent, a condition in which hemodynamic instability would result on abrupt cessation of pacing. Because of the increased risk of serious consequences that patients may experience in the event of pacemaker malfunction, the chart should be labeled clearly in some manner (brightly colored sticker) that the patient is pacemaker dependent.

The underlying rhythm can be uncovered by reprogramming to VII at a rate of 30 to 40 bpm and recording the underlying rhythm. Whereas it is often helpful to decrease the pacemaker rate gradually to allow the native automatic focus to "warm up," an abrupt reduction in the paced rate will more accurately simulate the response to transient pacemaker malfunction. Decreasing the lower rate limit also can be achieved by applying a chest-wall stimulation device against the skin overlying the pocket. This device will deliver a train of painless stimuli mimicking a rapid heart rate (100–120 bpm) and temporarily inhibit the device. This usually works best when the pacemaker is in the unipolar mode rather than the bipolar mode.

Evaluation of Sensing Threshold

The determination of sensing threshold establishes the adequacy of the sensed amplitude of the R wave (and/or P wave). Sensitivity is a measure of how easily the pacemaker can "see" the R wave or P wave. Sensitivity values, expressed in millivolts per centimeter (mV/cm), may be selected with the programmer and range from 0.5 to 8.0 mV/cm. The greatest sensitivity is associated with the smallest numeric value in mV/cm, whereas the least sensitivity is associated with the largest mV/cm value. Each value represents a cutoff for the ability of the pacemaker to detect the height of a given intracardiac electrogram. For example, an R wave with an amplitude of 2.4 mV will be just missed with a sensitivity setting of 2.5 mV/cm. By changing the sensitivity to 1.0 mV/cm, the generator will sense any signal with an amplitude greater than 1.0 mV and be able to track the R wave of 2.4 mV. To establish the sensing threshold, sensitivity is decreased progressively (from 0.5 to 4.0 mV/cm) until the sensed signal is lost. The point at which that occurs is referred to as the *sensing threshold*.

Because the concept of sensitivity is difficult to grasp initially, an analogy is often helpful. Consider *sensitivity value* to refer to the height of a fence that blocks the view of objects (an R wave or P wave) on the other side. Although the heights of the objects are fixed, the height of the fence can be varied. By lowering the fence (from 4.0 to 0.5 mV/cm), the object can be brought into view (*sensed*); by raising the fence, it can be shielded from view (*not sensed*).

In VVI (or AAI) situations, the lower rate limit of the pacemaker is programmed to a value lower than the intrinsic rate before testing is begun because one wants to be able to see the native activity. If the patient's native ventricular rate is too low, the sensing threshold test cannot be carried out. If one begins with the most sensitive level (lowest number) and progressively decreases sensitivity, threshold is reached when pacing is first observed to occur (i.e., the native rhythm is no longer "seen").

In DDD applications, the atrial sensing threshold is tested by performing the same process: Threshold is reached when atrial pacing is first noted. To test the ventricular sensing threshold, the atrioventricular (AV) interval is lengthened to exceed the PR interval to allow the native QRS to be seen. The ventricular sensitivity then is progressively decreased from its most sensitive value until a ventricular pacing artifact begins to appear at the end of the expected AV interval. Because of the large R wave amplitude in most patients, R wave sensing will still occur even at the least sensitive setting, in which case the sensing threshold is recorded as being greater than this (i.e., >4.0 mV/cm). Typically, one will program in the sensitivity value that is closest to one half the sensing threshold value.

Evaluation of Capture Threshold

Capture threshold refers to the lowest pulse-output value (volts) associated with stable capture of the myocardium and thus allows determination of the lowest safe pulse output associated with greatest battery longevity. In contrast to sensing threshold testing, the lower rate limit of the pacemaker is reprogrammed to a value greater than the intrinsic rate before testing is begun. As in sensing threshold determination, most devices feature an automatic capture threshold test. Frequently, the pulse width is the variable that is decreased progressively until the loss of capture, although some manufacturers have automatic threshold determinations in which the pulse output is progressively decreased at a fixed pulse width. Pulse amplitude and pulse duration can be compared by noting that a doubling of pulse output will quadruple the delivered energy, in contrast to only doubling delivered energy when pulse duration is doubled.

In VVI applications, the ventricular capture threshold can be determined by progressively decreasing the pulse output in the graded settings or by progressively decreasing the pulse width until loss of capture. In DDD applications, the method of capture threshold testing depends on the state of underlying AV conduction. With intact AV nodal conduction, the atrial capture threshold test is carried out as follows: The device is programmed to the DDD mode with a lower rate limit set to about 20 bpm greater than the native sinus rate. The atrial pulse output is decreased in a stepwise manner until the loss of atrial capture occurs, which is signaled by the appearance of ventricular pacing at the programmed lower rate limit. The ventricular capture threshold is determined by programming the device in the same manner as for atrial capture testing but with the AV interval shortened to less than the PR interval. The ventricular pulse output then is decreased in a stepwise fashion until the loss of ventricular capture occurs. This will be manifest by the appearance of native QRS complexes.

In situations where AV conduction is impaired, such as second- or third-degree AV block, atrial and ventricular capture threshold testing is carried out in a slightly different manner. For atrial capture testing, the device is programmed to the DDD mode with the lower rate limit to 20 bpm greater than the sinus rate and with the shortest possible postventricular atrial refractory period (PVARP). The atrial output then is decreased in a stepwise manner until the observed occurrence of an irregular rhythm as a result of the occurrence of mixed AV synchronous and AV sequential pacing. Ventricular capture threshold testing is carried out by programming the device to DDD with the lower rate limit to 20 bpm greater than the native ventricular rate. The ventricular pulse output is decreased in a stepwise fashion until a loss of ventricular capture and heart rate slowing are noted. For situations in which the native ventricular rate is too slow or an underlying ventricular rhythm is not evident, the emergency VVI feature that most programmers have will allow for rescue pacing and will allow time to reprogram the ventricular pulse output to an appropriate value.

Because of the time required to attain a stable capture threshold following implant, one should probably not attempt to decrease either the atrial or ventricular voltage output until the initial follow-up visit at 3 months. At that time, usually the pulse output value is reprogrammed to at least twice the capture threshold value. Tables 10-2 and 10-3 summarize the steps necessary to perform both sensing and capture threshold testing.

TABLE 10-2. *Sensing threshold testing*

VVI
1. Program LRL to 20 bpm less than native ventricular rate and with highest ventricular output
2. Stepwise decrease ventricular sensitivity (low to high mV/cm)
3. Threshold = moment when ventricular pacing begins

DDD
Atrial
1. Program DDD with LRL 20 bpm less than sinus rate and with highest atrial output
2. Stepwise decrease atrial sensitivity (low to high mV/cm)
3. Threshold = moment when atrial pacing begins

Ventricular
1. Program DDD with LRL 20 bpm less than active ventricular rate, longest available AV, and highest ventricular output
2. Stepwise decrease ventricular sensitivity
3. Threshold = moment when ventricular pacing artifact can be seen at end of QRS or in ST segment

AV, atrioventricular; LRL, lower rate limit.

TABLE 10-3. *Capture threshold testing*

VVI
  1. Program LRL to 20 bpm greater than native ventricular rate
  2. Stepwise decrease in pulse output
  3. Threshold = loss of ventricular capture and sudden rate slowing.
DDD (with intact AV conduction)
  Atrial
    1. Program DDD with LRL to 20 bpm greater than sinus rate
    2. Stepwise decrease in atrial pulse output
    3. Threshold = appearance of ventricular pacing
  Ventricular
    1. Program DDD with LRL to 20 bpm greater than sinus rate and short AVP (AVI <-PR)
    2. Stepwise decrease in ventricular pulse output
    3. Threshold = loss of ventricular capture and appearance of native QRS complexes
DDD (with second- or third-degree AV block)
  Atrial
    1. Program DDD with LRL to 20 bpm greater than sinus rate and shortest possible PVARP
    2. Stepwise decrease in atrial output
    3. Threshold = occurrence of an irregular rhythm (due to mixed AV synchronous and AV sequential pacing)
  Ventricular
    1. Program DDD with LRL to 20 bpm greater than native ventricular rate
    2. Stepwise decrease in ventricular output
    3. Threshold = loss of ventricular capture and rate slowing

AV, atrioventricular; AVI, atrioventricular interval; AVP, atrioventricular pacing; LRL, lower rate limit; PR, onset of P wave to onset of QRS complex; PVARP, postventricular atrial refractory period.

Sensor Evaluation

In patients with pacemakers that have programmable rate modulation, it may be necessary to reprogram the variable pertaining to this feature. Presently, the available sensors include activity, minute ventilation, and oxygen saturation, or combinations of these. The manner in which the sensor is initially set up depends on the manufacturer, and one should refer to the manual to obtain guidance. Generally, one ascertains whether chronotropic incompetence is present at the time of implant, and this becomes the primary criterion for selecting this type of device. It always should be remembered that patients who are taking medications that have negative chronotropic effects often exhibit sinus node dysfunction that may benefit from the DDDR device.

If chronotropic incompetence is suspected but is minimally present, the device can be programmed to the DDD mode at the time of implant. When the patient returns for the 3-month follow-up visit, an inquiry into tolerance of mild to modest physical activity may reveal symptoms suggesting inadequate pacemaker rate response and prompt reprogramming of the DDDR mode. To verify this, it is useful to have the patient walk two flights down a stairwell and back and then to reassess the heart rate response on return to the examining room. This can be done with the rhythm strip or through telemetry. Changes in the sensor-driven upper rate limit can then be made based on clinical judgment.

Subsequent Follow-up

Usually, patients who are not pacemaker dependent can be scheduled for annual follow-up visits. More frequent visits may be necessary depending on whether high-sensing capture thresholds are observed at the initial follow-up visit or if historical and physical findings suggest a problem with the pacemaker pocket wound. Patients who are pacemaker dependent probably should have follow-up on a bimonthly basis.

Medicare has provided guidelines for pacemaker evaluation services that depend on the type of pacemaker implanted. With single-chamber pacemakers, the recommendation allows for two follow-up visits in the first 6 months following implant and then annual visits. For patients with dual-chamber pacemakers, follow-up is suggested twice during the first 6 months following implant and then biannually.

Transtelephonic Monitoring

Transtelephonic monitoring allows the pacemaker's battery status to be monitored. Basically, the patient keeps in touch with the pacemaker clinic on a routine basis every 6 to 8 weeks after implant by transmitting a brief rhythm strip; the magnet is applied and then removed before the end of the transmission.

Telephone transmission of a rhythm strip is a fairly simple procedure. Transmitting systems involve ECG electrodes attached to a small box. The leads can either be put on the chest or attached to the fingertips, and the electric signals are converted into sound waves that are transmitted over the telephone. A special receiver in the pacemaker clinic, which is usually hospital based but can be in a practitioner's office, changes the sound signals back into standard ECG form. Because the frequency response of the telephone is extremely high, a high-quality ECG signal, comparable to a routine rhythm strip signal, can be transmitted. Figure 10-3 demonstrates a patient using a transmitter placed against the chest. On the back of the transmitter are two ECG leads that must be in close contact with the patient's skin. Figure 10-4 demonstrates a patient using the fingertip electrode. If the patient has a bony chest or lacks the coordination required to hold the telephone receiver against the transmitter that is held against his or her chest, the fingertip electrodes are preferable.

Some types of telephone monitoring systems sense the presence of a pacemaker spike and place a deflection representing the spike on the ECG paper. This solves the problem of visualizing low-voltage pacemaker spikes, but it can create deflections representing a spike if a portion of the QRS complex is inappropriately sensed as a spike. From patients with no pacemaker in place (the telephone transmission was for arrhythmia monitoring), we have received rhythm strips with pacemaker spikes neatly placed in QRS complexes. Not all telephone transmitters are designed to measure accurately the pulse widths of pacemaker spikes from dual-chamber pacemakers. Figure 10-5 shows an example of a typical transtelephonic recording with and without the magnet.

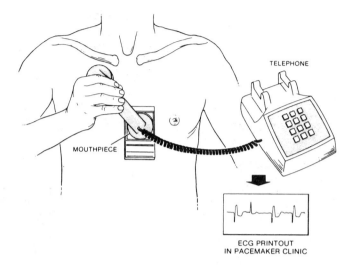

FIG. 10-3. Telephone rhythm strip transmitter. The patient is shown holding a battery-operated rhythm strip against his chest. On the back of the transmitter are two electrodes that are pressed firmly against the skin. These electrodes transmit an electrocardiogram, which is converted into sound waves and transmitted over the telephone mouthpiece to a receiver at the pacemaker clinic. The receiver then prints a rhythm strip.

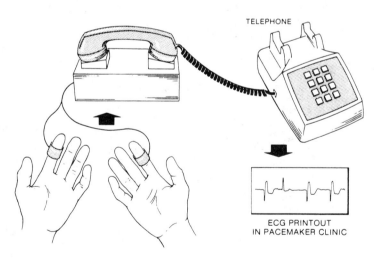

FIG. 10-4. Fingertip electrode transmitter. Electrodes are placed on two fingers and connected to a rhythm strip transmitter.

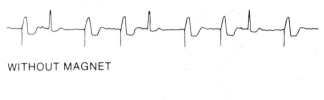

WITHOUT MAGNET

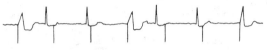

WITH MAGNET

FIG. 10-5. Typical pacemaker rhythm strip. This could be obtained from either a telephone clinic or an outpatient clinic. **Top:** The patient's rhythm without the magnet. In this example, the patient is in sinus rhythm followed by a pause, at which point the pacemaker begins to fire. Sensing is appropriate and capture is complete. **Bottom:** The magnet has been applied, and the pacemaker spikes march through the patient's rhythm without sensing the patient's intrinsic heartbeat. The second pacemaker spike does not capture because it falls within the patient's refractory period. (Note that we are using the term *refractory period* in the usual electrophysiologic sense, not as it is used in pacemaker terminology.) The first and fourth pacemaker spikes fall outside the patient's refractory period, and capture is identified. This represents normal pacemaker function. In this example, the magnet rate is the same as the paced rate, but in various models, the magnet rate may be slower or faster than the paced rate, or the magnet rate may change during the magnet cycle.

Diagnostic Considerations for Various Electrocardiogram Abnormalities

Lack of Capture or Intermittent Capture

In the case of intermittent or complete lack of capture, sensing may or may not be present. Figure 10-6 demonstrates a pacemaker that is neither sensing nor capturing. The differential diagnosis of this problem includes the following findings:

1. *Poor electrode position or dislodged electrode.* Occasionally, the electrode will not be firmly attached to the right ventricular apex and may "flip up" higher on the septum or out into the atrium. Less commonly, perforation of the myocardium or accidental placement of the electrode in the coronary sinus, rather than the right ventricular apex, occurs. Another cause of this type of malfunction is an epicardial screw-in electrode that has passed through the ventricle into the ventricular cavity and is not in good contact with the myocardium.

2. *Poor threshold.* Poor threshold may be present from the time of implantation, or a chronic rise in threshold, usually related to fibrosis around the tip of the lead, may occur. Less commonly, the patient could have a myocardial infarction involving the myocardium at the pacing tip, leading to a rise in threshold. Severe metabolic abnormalities can be a rare cause of noncapture. Cardiac medications such as antiarrhythmic drugs affect threshold only minimally and do not cause loss of capture unless the pacemaker is already functioning with a poor threshold.

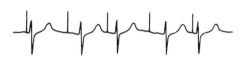

FIG. 10-6. Noncapture and non-sensing. A rhythm strip is shown from a pacemaker patient in whom the pacemaker is neither capturing nor sensing appropriately. The differential diagnosis of noncapture is discussed in the text.

3. *Lead fracture.* As a result of improvements in the pacemaker lead, nowadays lead fracture occurs fairly uncommonly.

4. *Poor connection between electrode and generator.* This problem is similar to lead fracture. Sometimes the pacing electrode has not been pushed far enough into the generator socket, or the set screw that tightens the electrode to the generator has not been tightened sufficiently. This problem usually occurs when a physician inexperienced at placing pacemakers is performing the procedure or when a new model is being used that is unfamiliar to the physician. Compatibility of the pacing electrode and the generator must be assured, especially if the two are not manufactured by the same company.

5. *Insulation break.* The Silastic or polyurethane coating around the wire may tear if too tight a suture is tied around the electrode during implantation. Another potential source of insulation break is improper placement of the insulating caps on top of the set screw. Breaks in insulation allow parallel electric circuits to occur in the system and may cause various pacemaker abnormalities.

6. *Battery failure.* At some point, a battery may fail and present with too low a voltage to capture the heart but enough voltage to generate a spike.

7. *Pseudomalfunction.* Lack of capture could be mistakenly diagnosed if it is not recognized that the pacemaker spike has fallen in the refractory period of the patient's cardiac cycle. This could occur if a magnet were placed over the patient's generator, thus disabling the sensing circuit, or if a sensing problem were present and the pacemaker spike occurred shortly after the patient's intrinsic QRS complex.

Total Lack of Pacemaker Stimulus

If an ECG tracing is obtained and no pacemaker stimulus can be detected when one should be present, some of the possible explanations include the following:

1. Total or nearly total battery failure.

2. Lead fracture or improper connection between the electrode and the pulse generator. In this instance, the resulting increase in resistance or impedance in the system is so great that no demonstrable electric activity is noted.

3. Complete inhibition of a demand pacemaker by skeletal muscle or electric magnetic interference. This problem is rare.

4. Lack of contact of the conducting plate of the unipolar pacemaker generator with body tissue during implantation. This situation generally causes confusion only during the immediate implantation of a unipolar pacemaker generator.

5. Pseudomalfunction. The incorrect diagnosis of lack of pacemaker stimulus can be made if the patient's pacemaker spike is quite small. Looking at multiple leads of an ECG tracing usually prevents misdiagnosis. The presence of hysteresis can cause confusion leading to misdiagnosis of pacemaker malfunction in a normally functioning unit.

Rate Change

Rate change is defined as a stable change in the pacemaker's rate of firing compared to the pacemaker's rate at the time of implantation. The differential diagnosis includes the following findings:

1. *Normal variation.* Minor chronic changes (1–2 bpm) in the pacemaker rate can occur in some patients. These may be related to the pacemaker battery and generator being exposed to body temperature for prolonged periods. Minor acute changes of rate can occur in response to fever. These changes are of no clinical significance.

2. *Battery depletion.* The most common cause for a marked drop in paced rate is battery depletion, especially in the mercury–zinc models. Pacemakers generally slow their rate in response to battery depletion as a sign that the elective replacement time is nearing. Information regarding the exact rate that indicates the generator should be replaced must be obtained from the manufacturer of the pacemaker.

3. *Inappropriate sensing.* If a pacemaker were to sense the preceding T wave consistently, it would result in a paced rate several beats per minute slower than the programmed rate.

4. *Random failure of a pacemaker component.* This is rare.

5. *Pseudomalfunction.* Incorrect diagnosis of an inappropriate change in pacing rate can occur if the patient's pacemaker is reprogrammed at a different rate but this reprogramming is not recorded. Malfunction of the ECG recording machine, with inappropriate paper speed, can cause misdiagnosis. Another potential cause for confusion is a pacemaker with a magnet rate that is slower than the pacing rate.

Intermittent or Erratic Prolongation of the Pacing Spike Interval

An example of intermittent or erratic prolongation of the pacing spike interval is shown in Figure 10-7. The differential diagnosis of intermittent or erratic prolongation of the pacing spike interval includes the following:

1. Sensing problems. Inappropriate sensing of the T wave, pacemaker afterpotential, or skeletal muscle activity can present this picture.

2. Intermittent fracture or poor electrode-generator connection.

3. Insulation break.

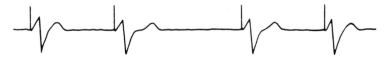

FIG. 10-7. Erratic prolongation of the pacing spike interval. This rhythm strip demonstrates an erratic prolongation of the interval between pacemaker spikes. The differential diagnosis of this rhythm strip abnormality is discussed in the text.

4. External electromagnetic or radiofrequency interference. This would be an unusual cause of malfunction.

5. Pseudomalfunction. Incorrect diagnosis can be made if hysteresis is misinterpreted as malfunction. An ECG recorder with a variable speed could create this picture. During telephone monitoring, a patient could accidentally or purposely wave a magnet near the pulse generator, causing variable pacemaker rate.

Lack of Appropriate Sensing

Figure 10-8 demonstrates a rhythm strip in which the demand pacemaker does not sense the preceding QRS complex appropriately. This differential diagnosis includes the following:

1. Poor electrode position or dislodged electrode.
2. Insulation break.
3. Battery failure.
4. Inappropriate programming of the sensitivity of the pulse generator. Obviously, this could occur only in pulse generators having programmable sensitivity or mode-of-response features.
5. QRS complex or broad QRS complex with a low slew rate. Bundle branch block with a low slew rate may cause pacemaker sensing problems. Occasionally, a premature ventricular contraction (PVC) will occur that, as detected by the pacemaker, is of too low a voltage to be sensed. Recall that the PVC seen on the surface ECG does not demonstrate the electrogram seen by the pacemaker.
6. Pseudomalfunction. Malfunction can be mimicked by the presence of an asynchronous pulse generator or a programmable pulse generator that has been programmed into the asynchronous mode. A PVC occurring in the refractory

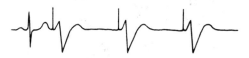

FIG. 10-8. Non-sensing. This rhythm strip demonstrates lack of sensing of a QRS complex. The differential diagnosis of this rhythm strip abnormality is discussed in the text.

period of the sensing cycle could be mistaken for a nonsensed QRS complex. A magnet held over the pacemaker converts the pacing mechanism to an asynchronous mode and could simulate improper sensing. Fusion and pseudofusion beats should not be misinterpreted as inappropriate sensing. The rarely used pacing mode VVT is a pacing generator that fires the pacemaker spike into the QRS complex and gives a confusing picture to those who are not familiar with VVT; it could be misinterpreted as improper sensing. Atrial pacing is present in three situations, two of which can cause confusion. Atrial pacing will, of course, occur in a DDD pacemaker at the lower rate limit. Sometimes atrial pacing occurs at a higher rate than the lower limit, and this is due to either (a) rate smoothing or (b) sensor-driven pacing. These are the only two situations in which a pacemaker paces in the atrium at higher than the lower limit. These situations do not represent malfunction. Generally, true malfunction also would involve a lack of atrial sensing.

Correction of the Diagnosed Problem

Although the preceding list is not complete, it does introduce the types of possible malfunctions that may occur with pacemakers and the patterns they produce on rhythm strips. The various methods of analyzing the pacemaker system that have already been discussed may have to be used to troubleshoot the pacemaker.

Correction of the problem, once it is diagnosed, may be effected by reprogramming the pacemaker, surgically exploring and changing the lead position, or replacing the lead or the pacemaker generator or both. The clinical status of the patient is of key importance in the clinical decision-making process. Some minor malfunctions may be ignored, depending on the clinical status of the patient. Patients have been known to receive a pacemaker that turns out to be unnecessary. Should such a pacemaker malfunction, simple removal of the pacemaker generator and lead (if removable) may be the best therapy.

Complications of Cardiac Pacing Unrelated to Electrocardiogram Abnormalities

Pacemaker Syndrome

Pacemaker syndrome is a symptom complex of lightheadedness, shortness of breath, or frank syncope that can be associated with hypotension, which develops or worsens after the initiation of cardiac pacing, usually ventricular pacing. Various mechanisms have been implicated in the development of pacemaker syndrome. These include lack of AV synchrony leading to decreased left ventricular filling and therefore decreased cardiac output. Syncope and presyncope have been seen and are thought to be associated with a vagal reflex that is initiated by elevated right or left atrial pressures caused by dissociation of the atrial and ventricular contractions. The atrium can contract against an already closed AV valve, thereby stretching the atrial baroreceptors and leading to a vagally mediated hypotension via a vasodepressor reflex. Also, "cannon V waves" can occur with ventricular pressure transmitted into the atria due to ventricular contraction simultaneous with atrial contraction with the valve open, and this can stimulate the cardiopulmonary baroreceptors to cause this reflex. Other symptoms associated with pacemaker syndrome include dyspnea on exertion, shortness of breath, and fullness in the neck along with pounding sensations or fullness in the head. These, in particular, may be associated with the cannon V waves, leading to elevated pulmonary capillary wedge pressures or elevated right atrial pressures. When the ventricle is paced directly, without AV sequential pacing, as pacing rates increase, further elevations of the pulmonary capillary wedge pressure, which can present as dyspnea on exertion, may be seen.

Most commonly in patients with pacemaker syndrome, there can be documented 1:1 ventricular-to-atrial conduction during ventricular pacing. Patients can have pacemaker syndrome in the absence of ventricular–atrial conduction; however, the most striking symptoms occur in patients with retrograde AV nodal conduction. Ideally, patients should be evaluated prior to selection to the proper pacing mode to check for this tendency. Institution of AV sequential pacing, when possible, is the best solution to this syndrome.

Stimulation of the Diaphragm

Stimulation of the diaphragm may be caused by perforation of the right ventricular wall by the pacing wire. Somewhat surprisingly, perforation can occur with few complications and is not by itself an absolute indication to change the pacing lead. Diaphragmatic stimulation also can occur without perforation of the right ventricular wall. One possible first step in correcting the abnormality is to lower the output by lowering the voltage in patients in whom this can be done safely. The pacemaker lead may have to be repositioned.

Pectoral Muscle Stimulation

Pectoral muscle stimulation usually is associated with unipolar pacemakers in which the electric current stimulates the chest wall muscles as it passes to the anode. With currently available unipolar pacemakers, this occurs less commonly because these pacemakers are designed to avoid concentration of a charge in one small area of the anode plate. If an insulation break were to occur (e.g., the insulators over the set screws are improperly placed or coming loose), current could flow in the area of the pacemaker generator and cause pectoral muscle stimulation, even in a bipolar unit.

Infection

Infection tends to occur shortly after implantation and to be localized, although endocarditis has been reported in association with pacemakers. Usually the pacing generator and lead must be removed to eradicate the infection, although cases have occurred in which the infection was treated successfully with antibiotic drugs while leaving the unit in place. The therapeutic approach taken depends on the clinical situation. Over a long period, the electrode often becomes fibrotic and difficult to remove from the right ventricular cavity. If the tip is fibrotic in the right ventricle, care must be taken because the heart can be pulled forcibly when the lead is pulled back, which may lead to severe arrhythmias. Prolonged gentle traction has been advocated to remove the lead in this situation.

If a patient with a pacemaker undergoes a procedure such as dental work that is likely to cause a transient bacteremia, the presence of a pacemaker per se is not an indication for antibiotic prophylaxis, probably because the pacemaker electrode becomes endothelialized with time. One (unproved) approach is to provide antibiotic prophylaxis in such situations only for the first few weeks after permanent pacemaker implantation.

Fortunately, pacemaker leads rarely need to be removed. Particularly, the tined leads tend to become embedded with fibrotic tissue and sometimes cannot be removed except by surgical intervention. If a lead is simply being changed without any complicating factors, an extra lead usually can be left in the heart without significant problems. Surgical extraction or, less commonly, light prolonged traction has been used to remove chronically imbedded pacemaker leads (see Chapter 9).

Erosion

Erosion of the pacemaker through the chest wall is a difficult complication to manage, particularly in persons with thin chests. Because modern pacemakers are smaller than the old ones, this complication is becoming less common.

Thrombosis

Thrombosis of the vein containing the lead occurs commonly but rarely causes clinical problems.

Patient Manipulation of the Pacemaker

Some pacemakers set loosely in the pocket. If a patient rotates the pacemaker beneath the skin either purposefully or absentmindedly, lead dislodgment or fracture can result. This is called *twiddler's syndrome*.

Runaway Pacemaker

Markedly inappropriate increases in pacing rate were a problem in early generators but are virtually nonexistent in current models. If such an event occurs, however, it can be life threatening. The treatment in a clinically unstable situation is to make a skin incision and cut the lead.

Lead Removal

Pacemaker leads rarely need to be removed. Particularly, the tined leads tend to become embedded with fibrotic tissue and sometimes cannot be removed except by surgical intervention. If a lead is simply being changed without any complicating factors, an extra lead usually can be left in the heart without significant problems. Catheter-mediated lead extraction is becoming more common, although the technique still is confined to a few tertiary care centers. Surgical extraction is rarely necessary.

Allergic Reactions

Allergic reactions to pacemaker coverings are rare.

Drug and Electrolyte Effects on Threshold

Many drugs can affect the pacing threshold, but most reactions are not clinically important. There are reports, however, that flecainide and encainide do raise the threshold significantly. Sotalol may possibly lower the threshold. A patient with end-stage renal disease may develop severe hyperkalemia, which in turn may lead to problems with both pacing and sensing.

Management of Clinical Problems in the Pacemaker Patient

Electrocautery

Surgery in the pacemaker patient seldom presents a problem, but electrocautery can cause sensing problems with pacemakers. If a patient with a permanent pacemaker requires surgery in which electrocautery is to be used, a consultant familiar with the patient and the patient's pacemaker and access to equipment to program that pacemaker should be available.

No standard method of handling electrocautery exists. Electrocautery should not be used within 6 inches of an implanted pulse generator. Bipolar electrocautery may minimize interference. If unipolar electrocautery is used, the indifferent electrode should be placed so that the current between it and the electrocautery site does not pass near the pacemaker or its lead. The minimal power setting should be used. Short bursts of power, spaced less than 1 second apart, will minimize any hemodynamic effects of inhibition. Placement of a magnet over the pacemaker converts it to an asynchronous mode, thus avoiding electric interference. We do not recommend this step, however, because the pacemaker may be reprogrammed as a result, but a pacemaker programmable to an asynchronous mode may be programmed in this manner. Decreasing the sensitivity of the pacemaker is not likely to be of major value because electrocautery is a powerful stimulus. If the electrocautery is likely to interfere with ECG monitoring during surgery, an arterial line may be used to document appropriate cardiac function during the procedure.

Basically, pacemaker manufacturers recommend that electrocautery not be used in patients with a pacemaker. If it must be used, consultation with a physician familiar with the patient and the patient's pacemaker and access to equipment to program that pacemaker should be available. The pacemaker company also should be consulted.

Electroconvulsive Therapy

A psychiatric patient receiving electroconvulsive therapy (ECT) may be handled in a manner similar to a patient having electrocautery; however, ECT is less likely to cause problems. The availability of a programmer, appropriate monitoring, and routine emergency equipment is the only requirement. The electric stimulus in ECT is far from the pacemaker.

Cardioversion or Defibrillation

A patient with or without myocardial infarction may require cardioversion because of supraventricular arrhythmia or ventricular tachycardia or defibrillation resulting from ventricular fibrillation. To minimize the risk of damage to the pacemaker when cardioversion or defibrillation is required, the lowest effective energy setting should be used. Another precaution is to direct the cardioversion charge being given across the chest wall in a direction perpendicular to the line between the anode and cathode of the pacemaker. This positioning will tend to send less electricity into the pacemaker generator. Usually, this is best accomplished by using anterior–posterior defibrillation paddles. (In other words, one paddle is placed on the front of the chest, and a flat paddle is placed beneath the patient's back.) The paddles also should be kept as far away as practical from the pacemaker generator itself.

Of course, in an emergency, the clinician should never be timid about shocking a patient who is hemodynamically unstable. The pacemaker could be repaired later if there is a problem, and fortunately there are rarely problems.

Hospital Bedside Telemetry after Pacemaker Placement

In a patient in the hospital with a pacemaker in place who is being monitored by telemetry (for example, to rule out myocardial infarction), the standard warning systems sometimes can be confused by the pacemaker. The most potentially serious problem is the development of ventricular fibrillation with pacemaker spikes still appearing. The telemetry warning system may interpret this as continued sinus rhythm and not alert the nursing staff to the possibility of cardiac arrest. Some sophisticated telemetry systems are designed to recognize this situation, but their reliability may be suboptimal. This is a greater problem with unipolar pacing; usually the bipolar pacing spike is too low to be monitored by the bedside telemetry.

Magnetic Resonance Imaging

Magnetic resonance imaging (MRI) subjects the patient to massive magnetic fields that will damage the pacemaker. Therefore, MRI studies are contraindicated in a patient with a pacemaker.

If MRI is absolutely required, consultation with the pacemaker company is warranted. It is of note that most pacemaker cases are made of titanium, and the case itself is not magnetic. MRI may inhibit the pacemaker, cause the pacemaker to pace asynchronously, or damage the pacemaker in other less predictable ways, such as causing a high rate or damage to the internal pacemaker circuitry.

When MRI is being considered, some theoretical concerns exist for a patient who has even a cut-off pacemaker lead in the heart. In theory, the powerful magnetic fields could create a small current in a lead, which could lead to ventricular arrhythmias. This, however, is more of a theoretic concern.

Anecdotally, we have heard of patients undergoing MRI after the pacemaker was programmed to VOO or DOO, without untoward events. Every case should be managed individually and the risk benefit assessed by the clinician at the bedside.

Radiation Therapy

Although x-rays from diagnostic radiography do not damage pacemakers, the high-energy ionizing radiation used in radiation therapy can damage the semiconductors of pacemakers.

Diagnosis of Myocardial Infarction

When a pacemaker patient has a myocardial infarction, the diagnosis can be difficult because of a completely paced rhythm distorting the QRS complex and T wave. Primary T-wave changes suggestive of acute myocardial infarction have been described, but cardiac enzyme elevation, along with the clinical picture, will allow the diagnosis to be made. Should an ECG be desired, some pacemakers can be programmed to a low rate and, assuming the patient's intrinsic heart rate is not too slow, the intrinsic QRS complex can be examined.

Lithotripsy

On the basis of preliminary reports, it appears that patients with transvenous VVI pacemakers in the thoracic position can undergo lithotripsy without major risk. It should be done, however, with cardiac monitoring and an appropriate pacemaker programmer available. If the pacemaker is likely to be directly in the beam of the lithotriptor, it is best to avoid this or to take special precautions. This situation is more likely to occur in patients who have the pacemaker in the abdominal position. There are also indications that a DDD pacemaker may be more likely to have problems with the lithotriptor, particularly the problem of inappropriate sensing in the atrial lead. Rate-responsive pacemakers also may have particular problems with lithotripsy. This is one of many situations in which the physician may want to consult with the pacemaker company ahead of time.

Cellular Telephones

Cellular telephones have been identified as a potential source of electromagnetic interference affecting pacemakers. This is actually a complex engineering issue. Analog telephones are more likely to cause problems than digital telephones, and within these categories various levels of interference are likely to occur. In general, however, digital telephones used reasonably are not a major risk. The general recommendations are to use the phone in the ear opposite the side of the pacemaker and to keep a 15-cm distance between the phone and the pacemaker. In particular, the phone should not be left in the "on" position in a pocket over the pacemaker. There is risk of electromagnetic interference with the cellular phones, but when used in a reasonable manner with the phone kept at least 15 cm away from the pacemaker generator (sometimes 30 cm for various models), cellular telephones do not cause a major risk.

Electronic Surveillance Devices (Antitheft Detector)

Stores more commonly now have electronic surveillance devices to detect shoplifters. The technology involved varies with the different companies making these. As is often the case, a detailed recommendation would depend on the exact device and the specific pacemaker. A general rule, however, is that if the patient with either an implantable defibrillator or pacemaker simply walks through the electric device without lingering and especially without staying within the electric field and turning around, the interference is likely to be minimal and of no clinical consequence. One problem is that these devices may not be apparent to the general public. The patient needs to be encouraged to lead a fairly normal life. We have heard anecdotally of one patient who would not enter any stores except through the back door and otherwise would leave the shopping to his wife. Such avoidance is being unduly concerned. At the same time, reasonable precaution should be taken to avoid the relatively rare situation of electromagnetic interference causing a problem when a patient lingers within the field of the electronic surveillance device. For example, when a friend tells a patient with a pacemaker to "meet me at the front door of a store," the pacemaker patient should be cautious not to linger within the field of an electronic surveillance device.

Complex Arrhythmias

Complex arrhythmias can occur as a result of pacemaker therapy. They are an uncommon development and, when they occur, they should be managed by someone knowledgeable about pacemakers and electrophysiology. Sometimes complex arrhythmias can be cured by changing the pacing mode or by manipulating the programmable features of the pacemaker.

Pediatric Patients

The pediatric patient presents a special difficulty in follow-up. Generally, the pediatric patient's problems are related to growth and subsequent fracture or dislodgment of the lead. The relatively thin wall of the myocardium in the pediatric patient represents a particular problem for the use of screw-in electrodes because the screw tends to go through the myocardium and leads to poor thresholds.

Pediatric patients often have problems with high thresholds, and safety margins may be of greater importance in this patient population. Follow-up through a clinic is generally required rather than just checking over the telephone.

Miscellaneous

At times, the patient may be exposed to powerful electromagnetic sources, and it is best to consult the pacemaker company involved for more details. Situations in this category include patients involved in arc welding, patients who are ham radio operators, and patients near a radar installation.

When a patient dies, pacemakers should be removed if cremation is being considered.

TEMPORARY PACEMAKER FOLLOW-UP

Troubleshooting malfunctions of temporary pacemakers is in many ways easier than troubleshooting malfunctions of permanent pacemakers. The connections are outside the patient and can be inspected easily. If any of the rhythm strip abnormalities described in the permanent pacemaker section occur, several possibilities exist. A wet sheet connecting two exposed terminals can cause a short circuit in the system. Examination should be made for any loose connections and to ensure that the pacemaker is turned on. Most cardiac care units keep close track of the battery life of pacemakers, but the possibility of battery depletion must be considered.

Fractures can occur in the pacemaker cable or pacemaker electrode, particularly if either has been resterilized several times. Intermittent fractures can be a frustrating problem to diagnose in temporary pacing situations. Sensing problems usually can be corrected by manipulating the switch on the temporary pacemaker labeled *asynchronous-demand*, which simply changes the sensitivity of the sensing circuit. The temporary electrode is a relatively stiff wire that can perforate the right ventricle fairly easily. Dislodgment of the temporary electrode is a more common problem than with permanent electrodes.

The temporary pacing system is more forgiving of poor electrode position because the temporary pacemaker contains an approximately 15-V power source, allowing the current to be turned up to as high as 20 mA in the temporary pacing system. This often allows cardiac stimulation, even if the electrode is in a poor position or if the threshold is high; however, this high current level often causes muscle stimulation of the chest wall that is uncomfortable for the patient.

Thrombosis formation in the vein containing the pacing lead can be a problem, especially in the femoral vein. Low-dose heparin or, if clinically indicated, full-dose anticoagulant drugs can be given to reduce the possibility of serious problems and generally is not associated with bleeding problems at the site of the pacemaker lead insertion.

REFERENCES

Altamura G, Gentilucci G, Santini M. Implanted pacemakers and cellular telephone interference. *Cardiology Review* 1998;15:38.

Bernstein A, Irwin M, Parsonnet V, et al. Report of the NASPE policy conference on antibradycardia pacemaker follow-up: effectiveness, needs, and resources (NASPE policy statement) (Part I) *Pacing Clin Electrophysiol* 1994;17:1714.

Blakeman BP, Wilber D, Olshansky B, Kall J. Coronary artery bypass in patients with previously placed implantable defibrillators. *Pacing Clin Electrophysiol* 1993;16:2087.

Brodell GK, Castle LW, Maloney JD, Wilkoff BL. Chronic transvenous pacemaker lead removal using a unique, sequential transvenous system. *Am J Cardiol* 1990;66:964.

Candinas R, Hagspiel KD, MacCarter DJ, et al. Premature ICD battery depletion due to a defective lead adapter component: usefulness of extensive data logging. *Pacing Clin Electrophysiol* 1993;16:2192.

Capucci A, Boriani G. Drugs, surgery, cardioverter defibrillator (Part II). *Pacing Clin Electrophysiol* 1993;16:519.

Chang AC, McAreavey D, Tripodi D, Fananapazir L. Radiofrequency catheter atrioventricular node ablation in patients with permanent cardiac pacing systems. *Pacing Clin Electrophysiol* 1994;17:65.

Colavita PG, Zimmern SH, Gallagher JJ, et al. Intravascular extraction of chronic pacemaker leads: efficacy and follow-up. *Pacing Clin Electrophysiol* 1993;16:2333.

Ellenbogen K, Gilligan D, Wood M, Morillo C, Barold S. The pacemaker syndrome—a matter of definition. *Am J Cardiol* 1997;79:1226.

Espinosa RE, Hayes DL, Vlietstra RE, et al. The dotter retriever and pigtail catheter: efficacy in extraction of chronic transvenous pacemaker leads. *Pacing Clin Electrophysiol* 1993;16:2337.

Faust M, Fraser J, Schurig L, et al. Educational guidelines for the clinically associated professional in cardiac pacing and electrophysiology (NASPE/CAP educational guidelines position statement) (Part I). *Pacing Clin Electrophysiol* 1990;13:1448.

Fearnot NE, Smith HJ, Goode LB, et al. Intravascular lead extraction using locking stylets, sheaths, and other techniques (Part II). *Pacing Clin Electrophysiol* 1990;13:1864.

Feldman CL, Olson WH, Hubbelbank M, et al. Identification of an implantable defibrillator lead fracture with a new Holter system. *Pacing Clin Electrophysiol* 1993;16:1342.

Frame R, Brodman RF, Furman S, et al. Surgical removal of infected transvenous pacemaker leads. *Pacing Clin Electrophysiol* 1993;16:2343.

Furman S. Pacemaker and implantable cardioverter defibrillator electrocardiography. *Pacing Clin Electrophysiol* 1993;16:1943.

Furman S. Automatic mode change. *Pacing Clin Electrophysiol* 1993;16:2079.

Furman S. Pacemaker syndrome. *Pacing Clin Electrophysiol* 1994;17:1.

Furman S, Parsonnet V, Song S. The Bilitch registry (Part I). *PACE* 1993;16:1357.

Griffin JC, Schuenemeyer TD, Hess KR, et al. Pacemaker follow-up: its role in the detection and correction of pacemaker system malfunction. *Pacing Clin Electrophysiol* 1986;9:387.

Harthorne J. Implantable defibrillators, pacemakers, and electronic antitheft devices. *N Engl J Med* 1999; 340:1117.

Harthorne J. Theft deterrent systems: a threat for medical device recipients or an industry cat fight. *Pacing Clin Electrophysiol* 1998;21:1845.

Hayes D, Naccarelli G, Furman S, Parsonnet V, and the NASPE Pacemaker Training Policy Conference Group. Report of the NASPE policy conference training requirements for permanent pacemaker selection, implantation, and follow-up (NASPE policy statement). *Pacing Clin Electrophysiol* 1994;17:6.

Hayes D, Wang P, Reynolds D. Interference with cardiac pacemakers by cellular telephones. *N Engl J Med* 1997;336:1473.

Hayes DL, Vlietstra RE. Pacemaker malfunction. *Ann Intern Med* 1993;119:828.

Heldman D, Mulvihill D, Nguyen H, et al. True incidence of pacemaker syndrome (Part II). *Pacing Clin Electrophysiol* 1990;13:1742.

Marchlinski FE, Gottlieb CD, Sarter B, et al. ICD data storage: value in arrhythmia management (Part II). *Pacing Clin Electrophysiol* 1993;16:527.

McIvor M, Reddinger J, Floden E, Sheppard R. Study of pacemaker and implantable cardioverter defibrillator triggering by electronic article surveillance devices (SPICED TEAS). *Pacing Clin Electrophysiol* 1998;21:1847.

Muller-Runkel R, Orsolini G, Kalokhe UP. Monitoring the radiation dose to a multiprogrammable pacemaker during radical radiation therapy: a case report (Part I). *Pacing Clin Electrophysiol* 1990;13:1466.

Nowak B. Taking advantage of sophisticated pacemaker diagnostics. *Am J Cardiol* 1999;83:172D.

Roelke M, Bernstein A. Cardiac pacemakers and cellular telephones. *N Engl J Med* 1997;336:1518.

Romano M, Zucco F, Baldini MR, Allaria B. Technical and clinical problems in patients with simultaneous implantation of a cardiac pacemaker and spinal cord stimulator. *Pacing Clin Electrophysiol* 1993; 16:1639.

Schuller H, Brandt J. The pacemaker syndrome: old and new causes. *Clin Cardiol* 1991;14:336.

Sloman G, Strathmore N. Permanent pacemaker lead extraction. *Pacing Clin Electrophysiol* 1993;16: 2331.

Song SL. The Bilitch report. Part A. Performance of implantable cardiac rhythm management devices (Part I). *Pacing Clin Electrophysiol* 1993;16:814.

Song SL. The Bilitch report. Part B. Performance of implantable cardiac rhythm management devices (Part I). *Pacing Clin Electrophysiol* 1993;16:823.

Sulke N, Dritsas A, Bostock J, et al. "Subclinical" pacemaker syndrome: a randomised study of symptom free patients with ventricular demand (VVI) pacemakers upgraded to dual chamber devices. *Br Heart J* 1992;67:57.

Vassolas G, Roth RA, Venditti FJ Jr. Effect of extracorporeal shock wave lithotripsy on implantable cardioverter defibrillator. *Pacing Clin Electrophysiol* 1993;16:1245.

Zuckerman B, Shein M. Cardiac pacemakers and cellular telephones. *N Engl J Med* 1997;337:1006.

Glossary

active fixation lead   An atrial or ventricular pacing lead with a screw-in tip to secure it actively to the myocardium at the time of implant.

acute threshold   The threshold measured at the time of initial implantation, usually the lowest threshold that will be obtained in the pacemaker's history.

after-potential   The small current present in the system after the pacemaker spike is turned off.

ampere   The unit of electrical current. It represents a charge moving at the rate of 1 coulomb per second. It is often abbreviated *amp* or *A*. Because the current in a pacemaker is low, the units are usually in thousandths of an ampere, or milliamperes (mA). Current is abbreviated *i* or *I*.

ampere-hour (Ah)   The unit reflecting battery capacity. *Ah* indicates that a pacemaker battery can deliver 1 ampere over a 1-hour period. Usually, the smaller the pacemaker, the lower the Ah value. The usual range is 0.8–2.5 Ah.

anode   (1) The positive pole of the pacemaker circuit. In bipolar circuits, the tip of the electrode is usually negative, and the more proximal electrode (the band electrode or ring electrode) is usually positive, although the polarities are sometimes reversed. In unipolar circuits, the tip of the electrode is usually negative, and the metal plate of the pacemaker wall itself is hooked to the positive end and thus is called the *anode*. The pacemaker will function if the polarities are reversed, but this is rarely done and may result in a higher threshold. (2) Within the battery, the anode is the material that gives off electrons. In the lithium iodine battery, the anode is the lithium. This is the less common use of the term *anode* in pacing literature.

antitachycardia pacing (ATP)   Using rapid pacing as described in the text to terminate a tachyarrhythmia.

artifact   (1) An ECG recording malfunction resembling an arrhythmia or pacemaker problem. (2) The small recorded mark or spike representing the pulse generator's electric output.

asynchronous mode   A pacemaker response in which the pacemaker fires independently of a patient's heart rhythm; therefore, no sensing occurs.

atrial escape interval (AEI)   The period in a dual-chamber pacemaker's timing cycle initiated by a ventricular sensed or paced event and ending with the next atrial paced event. Also known as the *VA internal.*

atrial refractory period   The atrial timing cycle during which the atrial sense amplifier is unresponsive to signals. In dual-chamber pacing modes, the total atrial refractory period comprises of the AV interval and the postventricular atrial refractory period.

atrial tracking   A pacing mode in which atrial contraction is sensed and the pacemaker will follow atrial contraction with a properly timed ventricular spike (or possibly be suppressed if AV conduction is intact and the ventricular portion of the pacemaker senses a normally conducted ventricular beat). This maintains atrial and ventricular synchrony to allow optimal cardiac output. If the patient has a normal atrial response to exercise and stress, it will allow rate responsiveness also.

AV interval (AVI)   In a dual-chamber pacemaker, the interval between an atrial event (sensed or paced) and the paced ventricular event.

AV interval extension   A prolongation of the AV interval caused by delaying the ventricular output pulse until the maximum tracking rate is reached. This occurs only in VDD or DDD modes and when the intrinsic atrial rate exceeds the programmed value of the maximum tracking rate.

bipolar   A pacemaker generator in which both the positive and negative poles of the circuit are in the area of the myocardium. A transvenous bipolar lead contains a wire leading to the tip electrode and another wire leading to the band electrode approximately 1 cm back. A bipolar transthoracic unit would have two myocardial leads, and electricity would travel from one to the other.

biphasic   A waveform morphology having both a positive and negative value.

BOL   An abbreviation for *beginning of life*, which refers to the pacemaker's battery status at the time of implant.

BPEG   An abbreviation for the British Pacing and Electrophysiology Group, a subdivision of the British Cardiac Society.

blanking period   An interval of time during which the pacemaker is unable to sense (or does not respond to sensed events). A feature of a noncommitted dual-chamber pacing system that helps avoid cross-talk. For several milliseconds during and after the atrial system spike, the ventricular system will not be inhibited by electrical activity (the blanking period), thus avoiding inappropriate inhibition of the ventricular system by the atrial system.

burst pacing   A method of pacing used to terminate a tachycardia. Several sequential, rapid, electric stimuli are applied to the heart in an effort to break up circus arrhythmia. This is a common way to interrupt atrial flutter, although it can lead to atrial fibrillation.

cadmium nickel oxide battery   A type of battery, rarely used now, that is externally rechargeable.

capacitor   A device made of two conductors separated by an insulator that is used to store electric charges until they are needed.

capture   The ability of the electric discharge of the pacemaker to initiate a propagated wave of excitation.

cardioversion   Restoration of sinus rhythm by delivering a synchronized low-energy shock or pulse. The shock is synchronized with the QRS complex to reduce the chance of ventricular tachycardia fibrillation, with the shock being on the T wave.

cathode   (1) The negative pole of the pacing circuit. In both the unipolar and bipolar systems, it is usually the distal electrode. (2) In battery terminology, the cathode is the material that takes up electrons. In the lithium iodine battery, the cathode is the iodine. This is the less common use of the term *cathode* in pacing literature.

chronaxie   The threshold pulse width on the strength-duration curve at twice the rheobase value expressed in volts.

chronic threshold   The threshold of a pacing system that has been in place for some time and is usually higher than the acute threshold.

chronotropic incompetence   The inability of the heart to regulate its rate appropriately in response to physiologic stress. This term usually refers to the lack of ability to increase heart rate in the normal way.

CMOS   Abbreviation for *complementary metallic oxide semiconductor*, a form of semiconductor often used in pacemaker technology.

coaxial lead   A bipolar pacing lead in which one helical conductor is wrapped around and insulated from the other coiled conductor. Coaxial leads are thinner than bipolar side-by-side leads. Also known as an *inline lead.*

committed ICD   An ICD that will shock the patient as soon as it is charged up, is in contrast to an ICD with "reconfirmation," which will double-check and ensure that the patient is still in the tachyarrhythmia before delivering the shock.

committed pacemaker   A type of dual-chamber pacemaker in which the ventricular system is committed to fire once the atrial system fires. Even if a premature ventricular contraction (PVC) occurs after the atrial lead has fired, the PVC will not be sensed, and the ventricular system will fire into the PVC. The design is particularly useful in a dual-chamber system with unipolar leads to prevent cross-talk (inappropriate inhibition of the ventricular system by the atrial firing) between the atrial and ventricular systems.

conductor A material with a fairly large number of free electrons that therefore passes an electric current well.

connector The portion of the pacing lead that is connected to the pacemaker generator. Examples of clinical problems involving the connector are poor insulation of this connection with the generator and poor contact between the generator and the connector.

constant-current pacemaker A pacemaker designed to provide a constant current despite variations in impedance. As impedance rises, voltage is increased to maintain a constant current. The increase in voltage is limited by the voltage capacity of the pacemaker.

constant-voltage pacemaker A type of pacemaker in which the voltage remains constant throughout the pacemaker's spike.

coulomb The unit of charge. It is either positive or negative. One negative coulomb represents the charge of approximately 6.24×10^{18} electrons.

cross-talk In a dual-chamber pacing system with atrial and ventricular pacing and ventricular sensing, the atrial pacemaker spike or its after-potential could be sensed by the ventricular system and inhibit ventricular firing. (The ventricular system might interpret the atrial event as a ventricular contraction.) This occurrence is referred to as *cross-talk,* and pacemakers are designed to avoid cross-talk using various methods. Cross-talk is more likely to occur if the atrial lead is unipolar (because of the large spike and after-potential) than if it is bipolar.

cross-talk detection window (CDW) A short timing cycle occurring immediately after the ventricular blanking period in some DDD pacemakers that alters the usual response to a ventricular sensed event. Any event sensed during the CDW results in a triggered ventricular output at the end of an abbreviated AV interval and is referred to as *ventricular safety pacing.*

current density A term referring to the degree of concentration of current used to stimulate the myocardium. For example, a large-tipped electrode has a lower current density than a small-tipped electrode with the same current because, with a small electrode, the current is concentrated in a smaller volume. The smaller electrode will stimulate the myocardium more effectively.

cycle length A general term in pacing used for the interval between any one type of event and the next event of the same type, usually expressed in millisecond. By dividing cycle length into 60,000, the rate can be obtained. (See Appendix I.)

demand mode A pacemaker unit that will sense electric activity in the heart and fire only when the patient's heart activity falls below a specified rate.

defibrillation threshold (DFT)   The minimum energy output associated with successful defibrillation. It is not as concrete a number as pacing threshold but is more a "probability" number.

diaphragmatic stimulation   Electric activation of the diaphragm by the pacemaker. The abrupt diaphragmatic contraction is noted clinically as hiccups associated with each pacing stimulus and occurs by indirect stimulation of the phrenic nerve (or directly in cases of perforation). It is most commonly seen in cases of lateral misplacement of the atrial lead.

elective replacement time (ERT)   The point in the pulse-generator service life at which the manufacturer recommends pulse-generator replacement because battery depletion had reached a point where system failure is likely to occur within 3 to 6 months. The ERT is usually indicated by a change in the magnet rate or the mode of pacing function.

electrode   The portion of the pacing lead that is exposed metal and transmits electricity to the body.

electrogram   The QRS signal as seen by the pacemaker. This will be of a different shape and voltage than any signal seen on the surface ECG.

electrolyte   In battery terminology, the electrolyte is the ionic conductor that separates the anode and cathode of the battery.

electromagnetic interference (EMI)   The miscellaneous radiofrequency waves from the environment that might affect a pacemaker.

endless loop arrhythmia   *See* pacemaker-mediated tachycardia.

end-of-life (EOL) indicator   A signal from a pacemaker that the battery is becoming depleted. Most commonly, the overall pacing rate slows to indicate that the battery is running down. The timing of appearance of the EOL indicator may be somewhat arbitrary. If, for example, the EOL indicator begins to become apparent at 3.2 V in a 5V pacemaker, the pacemaker may not be near the EOL if the threshold is very low chronically, or loss of capture could occur earlier if the chronic threshold is unusually high.

escape interval   The period, measured in milliseconds, between a sensed cardiac event and the next pacemaker output pulse.

event counter   A feature of some advanced pacing systems that provides a numeric count of certain types of predefined cardiac events: AR (paced atrial, sensed ventricular), AV (paced atrial, paced ventricular), PR (sensed atrial, sensed ventricular), PV (sensed atrial, paced ventricular), the percentage of time paced, and others.

event marker   A real-time annotation of paced and sensed events for a pacemaker, usually displayed on a programmer screen or ECG machine in conjunction with a simultaneously recorded surface ECG.

exit block   A nonspecific term indicating a high stimulation threshold leading to noncapture of the pacemaker spike; this term is rarely used now.

Fourier series   The set of pure frequencies that, when combined, represent a complex signal. In pacing, the pacemaker may sense the largest harmonics contained within the QRS complex.

Frank–Starling relationship   The relationship between filling pressure of the left ventricle and cardiac output or stroke volume. The higher the filling pressure, within limits, the greater the cardiac output.

fusion beat   A QRS complex that has been formed by depolarization of the myocardium initiated by both the pacemaker spike and the patient's intrinsic heartbeat.

heart block   Inappropriate terminology usually referring to AV block. The term should be avoided.

hermeticity   The term, as used in the pacemaker industry, refers to a very low rate of helium gas leakage from the sealed pacemaker container. This reduces the chance of fluid entering the pacemaker generator and causing damage.

housekeeping current   The amount of current used by the pulse generator even when it is not delivering an output pulse. A pulse generator uses a certain minimum current to maintain active circuits (sensing). It is usually measured in microamperes and is also known as *standby current*.

hybridization   The process of combining semiconductor chips with other components, such as resistors and capacitors, to form a single complex circuit.

hysteresis   An occasionally used response pattern in a demand pacemaker such that the pacemaker will not begin to fire until the patient's heart rate falls below a certain rate; but when the pacemaker begins firing, it fires at a rate that is faster than the escape rate.

impedance   A complex quantity having the dimensions of ohms. Whereas *resistance* applies only to idealized circuits with constant voltage and current and no capacitors, *impedance* is the proper term for the opposition to current flow in the pacing system. Complex mathematic methods exist for computing impedance, but for our purposes, Ohm's law is adequate to describe the relationship among current, voltage, and impedance. In this text, the terms *impedance* and *resistance* are used interchangeably, and the abbreviation R is used for both.

insulator   A material with few free electrons that therefore passes an electric current poorly.

internal resistance   A property of lithium iodine batteries such that the solid lithium iodide, which is a product of the reaction between lithium and iodine, separates the lithium and the iodine and eventually causes the voltage of the battery to drop, even though total chemical depletion of the lithium and the iodine has not occurred.

interval The period of time, measured in milliseconds, between any two designated cardiac events. In pacing, intervals are more useful measurements than rate because pacemaker timing is based on intervals, not rate. Numerous intervals exist and are outlined in Chapter 5 and in the pacing paradigms in Appendix II.

IS-I Abbreviation for international standard I for pacemaker connectors (see Chapter 2).

isoelectric line The flat line on an ECG indicating the period when there is no recordable electrical activity.

joule (J) The fundamental unit of work or energy. In electric terms, in the pacing system, the energy released can be expressed by the relation: voltage current × time = energy (in joules).

large-scale integration (LSI) A nonspecific term referring to the technology that produces high-density circuits having thousands of components in an area of a few square millimeters.

lead The portion of the pacing system that contains the wire with insulation, the exposed electrode tips, and a connector to connect to the generator.

magnet rate The predetermined rate at which a pacemaker will pace in an asynchronous manner when a magnet has been applied over the generator. The value of the magnet rate is related to the battery status such that a decrease in the magnet rate to a critical value indicates replacement time.

maximum tracking rate A programmable value in dual-chamber sensing and tracking modes (VDD, VDDR, DDD, DDDR) that determines the highest ventricular pacing rate that can be achieved in response to atrial sensed events with 1 to 1 AV synchrony at the programmed AV interval. Also known as *upper rate limit*.

mode The type of pacemaker response to the patient's intrinsic heartbeat. The three commonly used modes are asynchronous, demand, and triggered. The pacing mode is designated by the NBG code.

mode switching This is a programmable program in a DDD pacemaker to reduce the risk of inappropriately rapid ventricular response caused by a supraventricular arrhythmia. For example, if the pacemaker senses that the patient has gone into rapid atrial fibrillation, rather than track the fibrillatory waves with a rapid ventricular response, the pacemaker can switch automatically to a ventricular paced rhythm at a predetermined, physiologically reasonable rate without tracking the rapidly beating atrium. It then can automatically switch back to atrial tracking once the supraventricular tachycardia is terminated.

NASPE Abbreviation for the North American Society of Pacing and Electrophysiology.

NBG code NBG is a consolidated abbreviation for NASPE and BPEG. It consists of a three- to five-letter code designating the pacing mode devised and is periodically updated. The NBG code is universally used to describe the basic functions of the pacemaker and is described in greater detail in Chapter 5. The code was previously known as the *ICHD code.*

NIPS Noninvasive programmed stimulation, a feature of certain pacemakers that allows the implanted device to be used for repeated electrophysiologic testing in the patient.

noise sensing The ability of a pacemaker to sense electromagnetic interference from the environment and to identify it as such, therefore not responding inappropriately as if it were sensing a QRS complex.

nominal settings The settings of a pulse generator's programmable parameters at BOL. Nominal values also may be used to describe those programmable pacing parameter values that will safely pace most patients.

ohm (Ω) The unit of resistance; 1 ohm is the resistance that results in a current of 1 ampere when a potential of 1 volt is placed across the resistance.

Ohm's law Voltage (V) is equal to current (i) times resistance (R): $V = iR.$

overdrive pacing A method of suppressing a tachycardia with a pacemaker. The patient's heart is paced at a rate faster than the intrinsic rhythm. Sometimes this can interrupt a tendency to a circus arrhythmia and eliminate a tachycardia.

oversensing Detection by the pulse generator's sense amplifier of inappropriate electric signals (such as myopotentials, electromagnetic interference, T waves, or cross-talk between atrial and ventricular channels in DDD pacemakers). The oversensed signal may or not be visible on the surface ECG. Oversensing also can be referred to as *underpacing.* It is usually corrected by making the pacemaker less sensitive (increasing the mV value), programming to a triggered mode, or the judicious programming of the refractory period.

pacemaker-dependent patient A patient who needs a pacemaker to maintain proper cardiac rhythm to sustained adequate cardiac output sufficient for the activities of daily living. Such a patient may have little or no underlying intrinsic ventricular rhythm. Patients who have undergone AV junctional ablation are such patients.

pacemaker-mediated tachycardia (PMT) A tachycardia in which a dual-chamber pacemaker is part of the circus rhythm. The lead from the atrium senses, causing the lead to the ventricle to pace as part of a "macrocircus" rhythm. This can occur only with a VDD or DDD pacemaker, which senses in the atrium and paces in the ventricle. The most common example of this is retrograde atrioventricular conduction: Sensing of the atrial contraction causes ventricular stimulation followed by retrograde atrioventricular conduction, thus completing the endless loop or circus arrhythmia. The arrhythmia can be interrupted if the retrograde atrioventricular conduction is interrupted or if sending of the retrograde P wave can be blocked.

pacemaker syndrome A term referring to episodes of weakness and dizziness in a patient during paced rhythm. This is generally due to loss of atrial kick or simultaneous contraction of the atrium and ventricles as a result of loss of AV synchrony.

pacing system analyzer (PSA) An external pacemaker that is capable not only of pacing the heart during implantation of a permanent pacemaker lead or generator change but also of measuring voltage and current threshold, impedance of the system, and the amplitude of the sensed QRS complex. Some pacing system analyzers can be used to test a generator. Others may become capable of measuring slew rate and printing out an electrogram of the sensed QRS complex.

phantom programming A term referring to inadvertent reprogramming of a pacemaker due to electromagnetic interference from the environment (a very rare occurrence). A common example is associated with the use of radiofrequency current (catheter ablation or during surgery).

polarization resistance The resistance to flow of electric current that is brought about by electric current flowing from a metal through an electrolyte bath and back to a metal. It is caused by polarization of positive ions moving toward the negative electrode and negative ions moving toward the positive electrode. It is a time-dependent phenomenon, and the resistance rises as more ions migrate.

polyurethane A polymer used as an insulating material on a lead. Compared with silicone, it allows a thinner lead and is also slippery when moist, a helpful attribute when placing two leads in a small vein. Small, superficial cracks have been noted to occur on the surface with time, known as *environmental stress cracking.*

postventricular atrial refractory period (PVARP) The period after a ventricular beat (whether sensed or paced) in which there is no sensing in the atrium. This is critically important so that neither the ventricular beat nor its repolarization (T wave) is sensed as an atrial event accidentally. In addition, the atrial refractory period will not allow the sensing of atrial activity within the time interval of the programmed PVARP. This refractory period varies, but the longer the refractory period, the lower the allowable upper rate limit.

programmability A characteristic of most modern pulse generators that allows one or more parameters to be adjusted noninvasively before, during, or after implantation. *Simple programmability* refers to one or two programmable features, and *multiprogrammability* refers to three or more programmable features.

pseudofusion beat A QRS complex formed by depolarization of the myocardium initiated by a patient's intrinsic heartbeat; however, a pacemaker spike is present that distorts the QRS complex. This can be a normal occurrence in pacemaker function.

pseudomalfunction Normal pacing system function that is misinterpreted as a pacing system problem caused by a recording system problem or an artifact. It also can refer to an unexpected behavior of the pacemaker that may appear to be a malfunction but really is not.

pseudopseudofusion beat An electrocardiographic superimposition of an atrial stimulus on the native QRS complex. The atrial output pulse cannot contribute to the ventricular contraction. Pseudopseudofusion beats can occur only in dual-chamber pacing modes and are most common in DVI.

pulse width (Also called *pulse duration.*) The width of the pacemaker spike in time. A typical permanent pacemaker pulse width is 0.5 msec; a typical temporary pacemaker pulse width is approximately 2.0 msec.

rate modulation The ability of pacemakers to increase the pacing rate in response to physical activity or metabolic demand. Rate-modulated pacemakers use some type of sensor other than sensing intrinsic atrial depolarization. Also known as *rate-responsive* or *rate-adaptive.*

rate-responsive AV delay A programmable special feature of certain advanced pulse generators allowing the PV interval (sensed atrial/paced ventricular) during atrial tracking to decrease progressively as the sensed atrial rate increases. Also known as *rate-adaptive AV delay.*

rate smoothing Gradual slowing or speeding of the pacemaker rate based on a percentage of a preceding cardiac interval. This mechanism is programmed into some types of pacemakers to reduce or smooth abrupt changes in paced rate, especially at the upper rate limit of dual-chamber pacemakers. Conversely, if a patient were to develop an ectopic atrial tachycardia, this programmed feature would cause gradual increase in rate rather than abrupt increase in rate.

reconfirmation ICD An ICD that will charge up (taking several seconds) and then recheck to be sure that the patient is still in a tachyarrhythmia. This is in contrast to a *committed ICD.*

reed switch A small, flat piece of metal within the pacemaker that, under the influence of a magnet, can bend and complete an electric circuit. This is one way of sending signals through the skin to the pacemaker.

refractory period   (1) In pacemaker terminology, this term refers to a brief period after either a sensed beat or a paced beat in which the sensing circuit does not sense (or, if sensing occurs, it does not cause inhibition); so the pacemaker will not inappropriately reset with the electric activity present (preceding QRS complex, preceding T wave, or after-potential). (2) In electrophysiologic terminology, this refers to the period after a QRS complex during which a stimulus will not cause myocardial contraction (divided into the *absolute* and *relative* refractory period).

resistance (R)   The opposition, present to varying degrees in all matter, to the flow of electric current.

retrograde AV conduction   This refers to impulse propagation from the ventricles to the atrium over the AV node. Depending on the timing of retrograde atrial activation in relation to PVARP, the event may or may not be sensed. Retrograde conduction over the fast AV nodal pathway invariably will be associated with VP intervals less than 200 msec, whereas retrograde conduction over the slow AV nodal pathway will exceed this value. Pacemaker-mediated tachycardia probably is associated only with retrograde conduction over the slow AV nodal pathway.

rheobase   The flattened portion of the strength–duration curve indicating the point at which increasing pulse width is no longer associated with the progressive fall in voltage. Rheobase indicates the voltage (pulse amplitude) at which capture will not be improved by an increase in the pulse width.

safety pacing   A mechanism available in certain dual-chamber pacemakers that forces a ventricular output when an event is sensed during a special interval (cross-talk detection window) following the ventricular blanking period. The purpose of safety pacing is to eliminate cross-talk inhibition.

semiconductor   A crystal (usually silicon) that is normally a nonconductor and that has had its crystal structure contaminated with other atoms, causing it to be a partial conductor.

sensing   The ability of the pacemaker to sense and respond to the electrical activity of the heart.

sensing threshold   The largest intrinsic atrial or ventricular signal, expressed in millivolts, that can be consistently sensed by the pulse generator sense amplifier. The sensing threshold is assessed by measuring the R wave or the P wave for ventricular or atrial sensing, respectively.

silicone   An organic plastic compound used as insulation on the pacemaker lead. It has been in use longer than polyurethane and has a well-documented track record of reliability. It does not become slippery when moist and requires a thicker coating than polyurethane.

slew rate   The rate of change of voltage in the electrogram (represented by *dv/dt*). Premature ventricular contractions often are not sensed because of their low slew rate.

source impedance   For a pacemaker to sense electric activity from the heart, the activity must be transmitted to the pacemaker. The impedance or resistance associated with sensing is the *source impedance.*

spike   The brief discharge of electricity put out by a pacemaker to cause stimulation of the heart. A typical length of time the battery is "turned on" in a permanent pacemaker is 0.5 msec and, in a temporary pacemaker, approximately 2.0 msec. On an ECG, this will show up as a sharp vertical deflection.

strength-duration curve   A graph relating threshold to the pulse width. A very narrow pulse width requires a relatively larger amount of voltage to cause myocardial stimulation, and a wider pulse width requires less voltage; however, increasing pulse width does little to improve threshold beyond a pulse width of approximately 2.0 msec.

T-shock   This term is used in testing an automatic implantable defibrillator. About a 2 joule shock on a vulnerable portion of the T-wave with an AICD can often induce ventricular fibrillation deliberately, in order to check the device and be sure that it will defibrillate the patient.

telemetry   The ability of a device to receive data. Unidirectional telemetry was a feature of early pulse generators that could be programmed but not interrogated. Bidirectional telemetry allows the device to both transmit and receive data.

threshold   The minimum stimulus required to cause excitation of the myocardium. This can be measured in various ways, such as the minimum voltage required at a given pulse width, the minimum current required at a given pulse width, or the minimum energy required to cause stimulation of the myocardium.

tilt   This describes the drop in voltage as a capacitor delivers a charge.

total atrial refractory period (TARP)   The sum of the atrioventricular delay added to the PVARP. The total atrial refractory period limits the maximum upper rate limit possible in a dual-chamber pacemaker.

triggered mode   A type of pacemaker response in which the pacemaker will fire when a beat is sensed. For example, the ventricular sensing and pacing pacemaker programmed to VVT will fire into any QRS complex sensed (this mode is not commonly used now), and if no QRS is sensed within a set period, it will fire.

underdrive pacing   Pacing at a rate slower than a tachycardia, which sometimes can interrupt and terminate a reentrant arrhythmia.

unipolar   A type of pacemaker in which only one wire travels to the heart. Electrons travel from the tip of this wire back to the anode, which is usually the wall of the pacemaker generator. Two poles are present in this circuit, but one wire is passed to the heart.

volt (V)   The unit of "electric pressure" or electromotive force that causes current to flow. Voltage can be thought of as a difference in potential energy between two points with an unequal electron population.

watt (w)   The unit of power that is the rate at which work is done. One watt is 1 joule per second or: voltage × current = watts.

Wenckebach phenomenon   (1) In routine ECG use, this is generally described as a progressive lengthening of the PR interval until an atrial beat is not followed by a ventricular beat. The following sinus beat usually is associated with a PR interval shorter than the last PR interval seen prior to the nonconducted P wave. This is also known as *Mobitz type I second-degree AV block.* (2) In pacemaker terminology, the patient with AV sequential pacing may develop a Wenckebach pattern at its upper rate limit as a mechanism for slowing the paced rate.

Suggested Reading

Pacing and Clinical Electrophysiology. Futura Publishing Company, Inc., 295 Main Street, P.O. Box 330, Mount Kisco, New York 10549.

This is a valuable journal dedicated to electrophysiology and pacing, published since 1978. Anyone involved with pacemakers should have access to this journal.

Appendix I

Conversion Chart

1 minute = 60,000 msec
1 second = 1,000 msec

To convert a programmed rate [pulse per minute (ppm)] to a timing interval, perform the following operation:

$$\text{time interval (msec)} = \frac{60{,}000 \text{ msec/min}}{\text{programmed rate (ppm)}}$$

or

$$\text{programmed rate (ppm)} = \frac{60{,}000 \text{ msec/min}}{\text{time interval (msec)}}$$

Appendix II

Pacing Paradigms

ABBREVIATIONS

AEI: Atrial escape interval. Time after a sensed or paced QRS allowed before pacing of atrium ensues (LRL minus AVI).

AVI: Atrioventricular interval. Programmed time at which, if QRS has not occurred after sensed or paced P wave, ventricular pacing will occur.

LRI: Lower rate interval. Slowest rate (measured in msec) allowed by the pacemaker before pacing [or lower rate limit (LRI), in beats per minute (bpm)].

LRL: Lower rate limit. Slowest rate in beats per minute (bpm) allowed by pacemaker before pacing.

MTI: Minimum tracking interval [also maximum tracking rate (MTR)]. Lowest time interval allowed for AV sequential sensing/pacing.

PPM: Pulses per minute.

PVARP: Postventricular atrial refractory period. Time after sensed or paced QRS that atrial sensor is "turned off" (disabled) so that there is avoidance of sensing QRS or T wave as being atrial activity. Also, avoiding sensing of certain retrograde P waves or rapidly occurring atrial activity.

TARP: Total atrial refractory period. AVI plus PVARP.

URI: Upper rate interval [also upper rate limit (URL)]. This can be defined in various ways:
1. The maximum rate at which an atrial-tracking, dual-chamber pacemaker can pace before 2 to 1 block occurs (60,000 msec AVI + PVARP).
2. An atrial pace-tracking, dual-chamber pacemaker can be *programmed* to an upper rate limit below the 2 to 1 block point. This would provide a Wencke-

185

bach phenomenon at upper rate. (If the pacemaker is programmed to *above* the 2 to 1 block point, the pacemaker will not track to the programmed rate.)

3. A VVIR pacemaker would have a defined upper rate limit in response to the sensor.

VRP: Ventricular refractory period. Time after a sensed or paced QRS during which ventricular sensing is effectively "turned off."

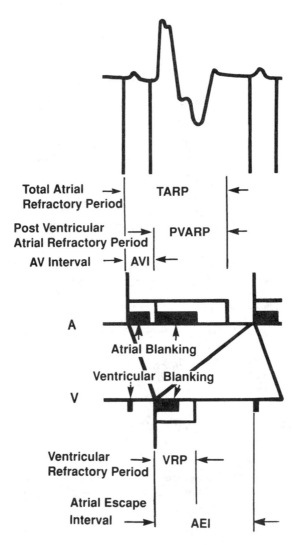

Ladder diagram of interval definitions.

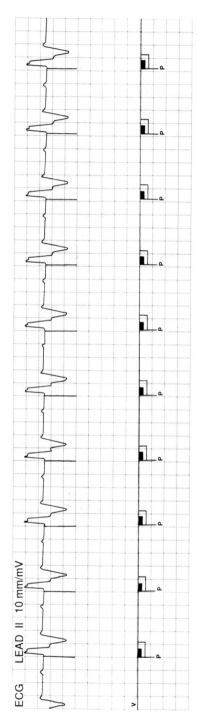

ECG LEAD II 10 mm/mV

VVI (A, atrium; V, ventricle; P, pace; S, sense; R, event occured during refractory period).

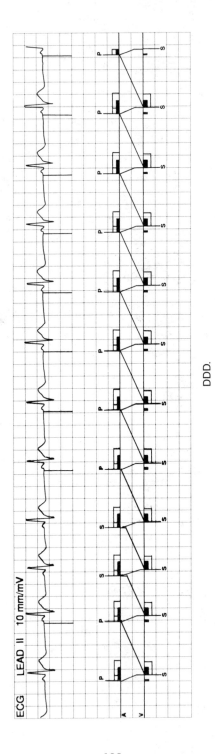

DDD.

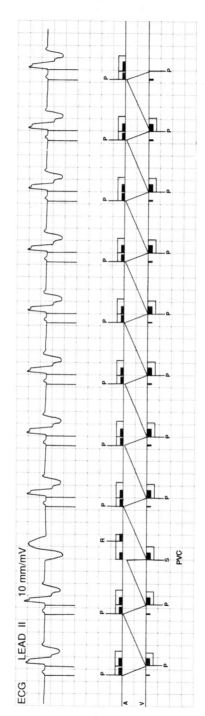

DDD with premature ventricular contraction (PVC).

189

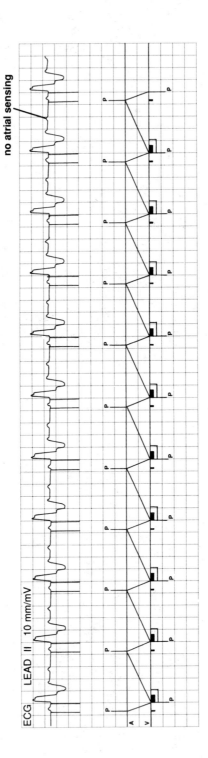

DVI.

190

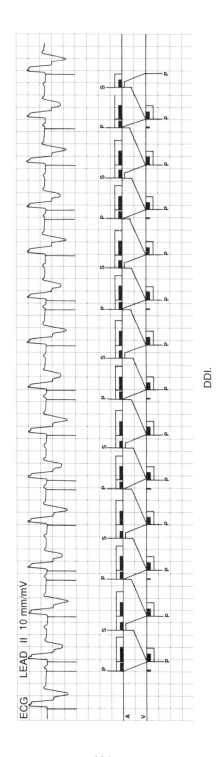

DDI.

191

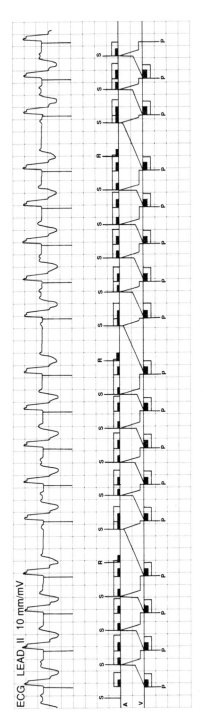

DDD with AV Wenckebach.

192

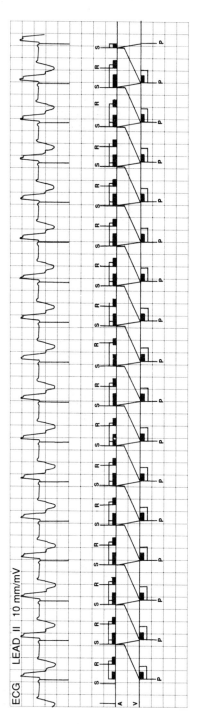

DDD with 2:1 BLOCK.

193

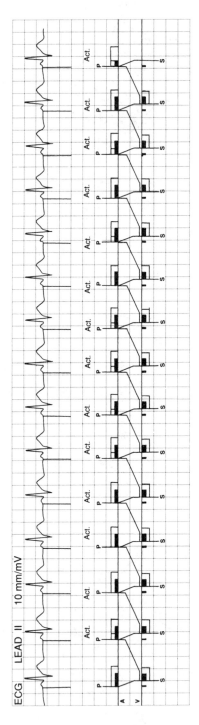

DDDR with chronotropic incompetence.

194

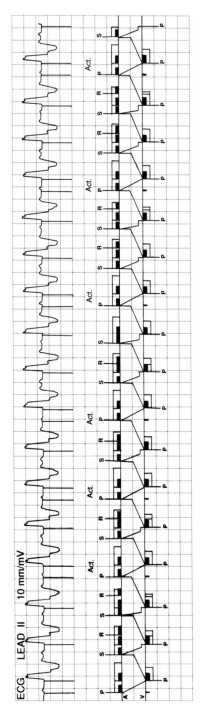

DDDR with competing sinus rate.

195

Subject Index

Note: Page numbers followed by f indicate figures; those followed by t indicate tables.

A

Accelerometer motion sensor, 104–105
Active fixation lead, 167
Acute threshold, 167
Afterpotential, 47, 48f, 167
Allergic reactions, 159
American Heart Association, 75–76, 77t
Amiodarone, 121
Ampere, 27, 167
Ampere-hours, 29, 167
Amplitude, in electrocardiogram
    recording, 56, 58, 58f
Anode, 167
Antitachycardia therapy
    implantable cardioverter defibrillator
        for, 111–123 (*See also* Implantable
        cardioverter defibrillator)
    pacing as, 167
    temporary pacemaker therapy for,
        21–22
Antitheft detector, 162
Arm veins, 140f
Arrhythmias
    complex, 163
    endless loop, 171
Artifact, 167
Asynchronous mode, 167
Atria, silent, 78
Atrial escape interval, 80, 168
Atrial flutter, 22
Atrial J lead, 34, 35f
    in transvenous implantation, 128
Atrial kick, 86f
Atrial pacing, esophageal pacing for,
    92–93
Atrial refractory period, 168
    total, 80
Atrial synchronous pacing, 81–82, 81f, 82f
Atrial tachycardia, 22
Atrial tracking, 168

Atrioventricular block
    complete, 6
    high-risk, 7–8
    His bundle electrogram in, 3–4, 3f
    infranodal, 6
    Mobitz I, 5, 7, 8
    Mobitz II, 5–6, 7
    with myocardial infarction, 17–22
        anterior, 18–21, 19f
        inferior, 17–18, 18f
    nomenclature of, 2–3
    pathophysiology of, 4–6, 4f
    permanent therapy in, 6–8
    second degree, 7
    third degree, 6
    transcutaneous pacing for, 92
Atrioventricular synchrony, 84–88
    cardiac output in, 86, 86f
    tachycardia decrease in, 86, 87f, 88
    valve closure in, 84
Atrioventricular valve closure, 84
Atropine, 137
Automatic mode switching, 99
AV delay, rate-responsive, 99
AV interval, 79, 79f, 168
    extension of, 168
AV sequential pacing, 81f, 82–83

B

Basic intervals. *See* Timing cycles
    (intervals)
Basilic vein, 140f
Battery
    cadmium nickel oxide, 31, 169
    failure of, 153, 154
    life of
        hysteresis on, 70
        pulse-width programmability on,
            63–64, 64f
        voltage programmability on, 65, 65f

Battery (*cont.*)
  lithium iodine, 29–31
  lithium vanadium silver pentoxide, 31
  of permanent pacemaker, 28–31, 28f
  of temporary pacemaker, 42
BBB. *See* Bundle branch block
Beta-adrenergic blockers, for syncope, 17
Bezold-Jarish reflex, 10
Bifascicular block, 19–20
Biphasic, 168
Bipolar, 168
  vs. unipolar pacemaker, 37–41, 37f–39f
Bipolar lead, 34f
  of temporary pacemakers, 42–43
Blanking period, 79, 79f, 168
BOL (beginning of life), 168
BPEG, 168
Bradycardia
  hysteresis in, 70–71
  and Mobitz II block, 7
  pacing for, 116
  symptomatic, 1
British Pacing and Electrophysiology
    Group (BPEG), 75–76, 77t
Bundle branch block, 20
  catheter placement in, 21
  high-risk, 7–8
Burst pacing, 116, 117f, 168–169

C

Cadmium nickel oxide battery, 31, 169
Capacitor, 169
Capture, 169
  lack of, 152–153, 153f
Capture threshold, evaluation of, 147–148,
    149t
Cardiac output, in dual-chamber
    pacemaker, 86, 86f
Cardiac standstill, 137
Cardiac surgery, temporary pacing after,
    140–141
Cardioinhibitor reflex, in hypersensitive
    carotid sinus syndrome, 12
Cardioversion, 169
  for atrial tachycardia, 22
  low-energy, 119f, 120
  as pacing abnormality, 160
  vs. defibrillation, 123

Cardioverter defibrillator, implantable,
    111–123. *See also* Implantable
    cardioverter defibrillator
Carotid sinus massage
  in head-up tilt table therapy, 16
  in pacemaker-mediated tachycardia, 97
Carotid sinus syndrome, hypersensitive, 12
Catecholamines
  in rate-modulated pacing, 105–106,
    106f
  on threshold changes, 53
Catheter
  for esophageal pacing, 92–93
  in transvenous temporary pacing,
    approach for, 88
Cathode, 169
Cellular telephones, 162
Cephalic vein, 127, 128f
Chronaxie, 169
Chronic threshold, 169
Chronotropic incompetence, 169
Circuit(s)
  electric, 28, 28f
  of permanent pacemaker, 31–33, 32f
  specialized, 61–73 (*See also*
    Programmability)
  unipolar, 43–44, 44f
Coaxial lead, 169
Committed ICD, 169
Committed pacemaker, 169–170
Complementary metallic oxide
    semiconductor (CMOS), 32, 32f,
    169
Conduction time, between SA node and
    atrium, 10
Conductors, 28, 170
Connector, 170
Constant-current pacing, 49–50, 50f, 170
Constant-voltage capacitor-coupled
    pacemaker, 49, 50f
Constant-voltage pacing, 48–49, 49f, 50f,
    170
Conversion chart, 183
Coulomb, 27, 170
Cross-talk, 170
  in dual-chamber pacing, 95–96, 96f
  in timing cycles, 79
Cross-talk detection window, 170

Current density, 170
Current threshold, 51–52, 52t
Cycle length, 170

D

DDD mode, 83–84, 85t
  with 2:1 block, ECG of, 193
  with AV Wenckebach, ECG of, 192
  ECG of, 188–189
DDDR, ECG of, 194–195
DDI mode, 83, 85t
  ECG of, 191
Defibrillation. *See also* Implantable
    cardioverter defibrillator
  as pacing abnormality, 160
  for ventricular fibrillation, 120
  vs. cardioversion, 123
Defibrillation threshold, 171
Deltopectoral groove, 127, 128f
Demand mode, 170
Depolarization, in His bundle electrogram,
    3–4, 3f
Device-device interaction, with
    implantable cardioverter
    defibrillator, 121
Diaphragm, stimulation of, 157, 171
Digoxin, for pacemaker-mediated
    tachycardia, 97
Discharge testing, of implantable
    cardioverter defibrillator, 122
Disopyramide, for syncope, 17
Drug-device interaction, with implantable
    cardioverter defibrillator, 121
Drugs, on threshold, 159
Dual-chamber pacing, 78–88, 95–100
  atrioventricular valve closure in, 84
  automatic mode switching in, 99
  cardiac output in, 86, 86f
  cross-talk and ventricular safety pacing
    in, 95–96, 96f
  DDI mode in, 85t
  modes of, 81f–82f, 85f
  pacemaker-mediated tachycardia in,
    96–98, 97f
  programmability of, 99–100, 100t
  rate-responsive AV delay in, 99
  tachycardia decrease in, 86–88, 87f
  temporary pacemakers in, 100

timing cycles (intervals) in, 78–80, 79f
  upper rate limit in, 98–99
  VDD mode in, 81f–82f, 85t
  VDI mode in, 85t
DVI mode, ECG of, 190

E

Elective replacement time, 171
Electric circuit, 28, 28f
Electrocardiogram(s)
  abnormalities in, diagnostic
    considerations for, 152–156, 153f,
    155f
  bipolar *vs.* unipolar, 38–40, 39f
  of DDD mode, 188–189
  of DDD mode, with 2:1 block, 193
  of DDD mode, with AV Wenckebach,
    192
  of DDDR, 194–195
  of DDI mode, 191
  of DVI mode, 190
  follow-up, 144–145, 144f, 145f
  of His bundle, in atrioventricular block,
    3–4, 3f
  minute ventilation on, 107, 107f
  QRS sensing in, 55–56, 56f, 57f
  recording of, 57f
  in transcutaneous pacing, 90–91, 91f
  transtelephonic monitoring of, 150,
    151f, 152f
  of VVI mode, 187
Electrocautery, 159–160
Electroconvulsive therapy, 160
Electrode, 171
  poor connection of, 153
  position, in lack of capture, 152
Electrode tip
  bipolar *vs.* unipolar, 40
  in permanent pacemaker, 41, 42f
  in polarization resistance, 47–48, 58
  porous, 58, 58f
  in transvenous temporary pacing,
    approach for, 88
Electrogram, 171
Electrolytes, 171
  on threshold, 159
Electromagnetic interference, 171
  noise-sensing circuit for, 66–67

Electronic surveillance devices, 162
Electrophysiology, of pacing, 47–59. *See also* Pacing, electrophysiology of
Emergency pacing, 136–137
End-of-life indicator, 171
Endless loop, 96, 97f
Endless loop arrhythmia, 171
Energy, programming output of, 72
Epicardial lead, 35, 36f
Erosion, 158
Escape interval, 171
Esophageal pacing, 92–93
Event counter, 171
Event marker, 171
Excitable gap, 116, 117f
Exit block, 172

F
Fascicular block, 20
Femoral vein, 137–138, 138f
Fibrous tissue, on pacemaker tip, 54
Follow-up, of pacemaker patient, 143–164
    capture threshold evaluation in, 147–148, 149t
    cardiac pacing complications in, 156–159
    clinical problems in, management of, 159–163
    ECG abnormalities in, diagnostic considerations for, 152–156, 153f, 155f
    electrocardiogram in, 144–145, 144f, 145f
    history and physical in, 143, 144t
    magnet rate in, 145
    pacemaker interrogation in, 146
    sensing threshold evaluation in, 146–147, 148t
    sensor evaluation in, 149
    subsequent follow-up in, 150
    temporary pacemakers in, 163–164
    transtelephonic monitoring in, 150, 151f, 152f
    underlying rhythm establishment in, 146
Fourier series, 56, 58, 172
Frank-Starling relationship, 86, 86f, 172
Fully automatic pacemaker, 83
Fusion beat, 172

G
Generator
    of implantable cardioverter defibrillator, 112
    of permanent pacemakers, 135–136
    of temporary pacemakers, 42
    of transcutaneous pacemakers, 90f

H
Head-up tilt test, 15–16, 15f
Heart block, 172
Hermeticity, 172
    of batteries, 29
His bundle electrogram, in atrioventricular block, 3–4, 3f
Hospital discharge, 122
Hospital telemetry, 160–161
Housekeeping current, 172
Hybridization, 172
    of circuits, 32, 32f
Hypersensitive carotid sinus syndrome, 12
Hypertrophic obstructive cardiomyopathy, 12–13
Hysteresis, 172
    programmability of, 70–71, 71f

I
Impedance, 27–28, 172
    source, 55–56
    in threshold determination, 53
Implantable cardioverter defibrillator, 111–123
    complications of, 122–123
    device-device interaction in, 121
    discharge testing of, 122
    drug-device interaction in, 121
    follow-up care for, 122–123
    future trends for, 123
    generator for, 112
    and hospital discharge, 122
    indications for, 111–112
    leads for, 112–113, 113f
    magnets in, 120–121
    system operation of, 114–115, 114f
    tachycardia detection in, 115
    and temporary pacemakers, 123
    therapy tiers in, 116–120, 118f–119f
Implantation, of pacemaker, 127–141

permanent, 127–136
  complication in, 133–135
  generator change in, 135–136
  lead and generator connection in,
      132, 133f
  perioperative care in, 133, 134f
  transthoracic, 129–131, 130f, 132f
  transvenous, 127–129, 128f
temporary, 136–141
  after cardiac surgery, 140–141
  emergency pacing in, 136–137
  transvenous, 137–140, 138f–140f
Infection, 157–158
Infranodal atrioventricular block, 4f, 6
  with myocardial infarction, 18–19, 19f
Insulation, break in, 153
Insulator, 28, 172
Intermittent capture, 152–153, 153f
Internal resistance, 172–173
International Standard I, 33
Interval, 173. *See also* Timing cycles
      (intervals)
IS-I, 173
Isoelectric line, 173
Isoproterenol, 137

J
J-lead
  atrial, 34, 35f, 128
  chest radiograph of, 134f
  in single-chamber atrial pacing, 88–89
Joule, 28, 173
Jugular vein, 139, 139f

K
Korotkoff's sounds, 16

L
Lack of capture, 152–153, 153f
Large-scale integration, 32, 173
Lead(s), 173
  active fixation, 167
  coaxial, 169
  fracture of, 152
  for implantable cardioverter
      defibrillator, 112–113, 113f
  myocardial placement of, 131
  of permanent pacemaker, 33–36,
      34f–36f

removal of, 159
  of temporary pacemaker, 42–43
Lenegre's disease, 6
Lev's disease, 6
Lidocaine (Xylocaine), for esophageal
      catheter, 93
Lithium iodine battery, 29–31
Lithium vanadium silver pentoxide battery,
      31
Lithotripsy, 161–162

M
Magnet rate, 145, 173
Magnetic resonance imaging (MRI), 161
Magnets, for implantable cardioverter
      defibrillator, 120–121
Maximum tracking rate, 80, 173
Measured data, 146
Minute ventilation (respiration), in rate-
      modulated pacing, 107, 107f
Mobitz atrioventricular block, 4–5, 7
Mode, 173
Mode selection algorithm, 87f
Mode switching, 173–174
  automatic, 99
Myocardial infarction
  anterior, atrioventricular block in,
      18–21, 19f
  diagnosis of, 161
  inferior, atrioventricular block in,
      17–18, 18f
  as pacing indication, 10–12, 11t
Myocardial lead placement, 131
Myocardium, voltage threshold of, 51

N
NASPE, 174
NBG code, 75–76, 77t, 174
NIPS (noninvasive programmed
      stimulation), 174
Nodal block, *vs.* infranodal, 4f
Noise-sensing, 174
  circuit for, 66–67
Nominal settings, 174
North American Society of Pacing and
      Electrophysiology (NASPE),
      75–76, 77t
Nuclear power, for pacemaker, 31

O

Ohm, 174
Ohm's law, 27, 174
Overdrive pacing, 116, 174
Overdrive suppression, 9
  for atrial flutter, 22
Oversensing, 174
Oxygen saturation, in rate-modulated
    pacing, 108

P

P wave
  in DVI mode, 83
  in emergency pacing, 137
  in His bundle electrogram, 3, 3f
  in pacemaker-mediated tachycardia, 96,
    97f
  in VDD mode, 81–82, 81f, 82f
Pacemaker
  battery of (*See* Battery)
  bipolar, *vs.* unipolar, 37–41, 37f–39f
  codes for, 75–76, 77t
  committed, 169–170
  constant-voltage capacitor-coupled, 49,
    50f
  dual-chamber, 78–88
    atrioventricular valve closure in, 84
    cardiac output in, 86, 86f
    DDD mode in, 83–84, 85t
    DDI mode in, 83, 85t
    special considerations in, 95–100
      (*See also* Dual-chamber pacing)
    tachycardia decrease in, 86–88, 87f
    timing cycles (intervals) in, 78–80,
      79f
    VDD mode in, 81–82, 81f–82f, 85t
    VDI mode in, 82–83, 85t
  electrophysiology of, 47–59 (*See also*
    Pacing, electrophysiology of)
  esophageal pacing with, 92–93
  follow-up for, 143–164 (*See also*
    Follow-up)
  fully automatic, 82f, 83–84
  implantation of, 127–141 (*See also*
    Implantation, of pacemaker)
  indications for
    permanent, 2–17
      atrioventricular block in, 2–8
      general guidelines in, 1–2
      hypersensitive carotid sinus
        syndrome in, 12
      hypertrophic obstructive
        cardiomyopathy in, 12–13
      myocardial infarction in, 10–12,
        11t
      sick sinus syndrome in, 8–10
      syncope summary in, 13–17, 14f
    temporary, 17–22
      antitachycardia therapy in, 21–22
      atrioventricular block with
        myocardial infarction, 17–21
  interrogation of, 146
  lack of stimulus to, 153–154
  leads of (*See* Lead[s])
  mode selection algorithm for, 87f
  patient manipulation of, 158
  programmability of, 61–73 (*See also*
    Programmability)
  rate of (*See* Rate; Rate-modulated
    pacing)
  runaway, 158–159
  single-chamber, 78
    transvenous temporary pacing with,
      88–89
  technology of
    permanent, 27–42
      basic principles in, 28
      circuitry in, 31–33, 32f
      electrode tip in, 41, 42f
      pacemaker lead in, 33–36, 34f–36f
      power sources in, 28–31, 28f
      term definitions in, 27–28
      unipolar *vs.* bipolar, 37–41,
        37f–39f
    temporary, 42–43
  transcutaneous temporary pacing with,
    89–92, 89f, 90f
  transvenous, 37–38, 38f
    temporary pacing with, 88–89
  unipolar *vs.* bipolar, 37–41, 37f–39f
Pacemaker-dependent patient, 174
Pacemaker-mediated tachycardia, 96–98,
    97f, 174–175
Pacemaker syndrome, 84, 156–157, 175
Pacing
  atrial, esophageal pacing for, 92–93

atrial synchronous, 81–82, 81f, 82f
atrioventricular sequential, 81f, 82–83
complications in, follow-up on,
    156–159
constant-current, 49–50, 50f, 170
constant-voltage, 48–49, 49f, 50f, 170
dual-chamber, 78–88 (*See also* Dual-
    chamber pacing)
  special considerations in, 95–100
electrophysiology of, 47–59
  constant-current, 49–50, 50f
  constant-voltage, 48–49, 49f, 50f
  polarization resistance in, 47–48, 48f
  sensing in, 55–58, 56f–58f
  strength-duration curve in, 52, 53f
  system impedance in, 53
  temporary pacing applications in, 59
  threshold changes in, 53–54, 54f, 55f
  voltage and current threshold in,
    51–52, 52t
esophageal, 92–93
implantable cardioverter defibrillator
    for, 111–123 (*See also* Implantable
    cardioverter defibrillator)
indications for
  permanent, 2–17
    atrioventricular block in, 2–8
    general guidelines in, 1–2
    hypersensitive carotid sinus
      syndrome in, 12
    hypertrophic obstructive
      cardiomyopathy in, 12–13
    myocardial infarction in, 10–12,
      11t
    sick sinus syndrome in, 8–10
    syncope summary in, 13–17, 14f
  temporary, 17–22
    antitachycardia therapy in, 21–22
    atrioventricular block with
      myocardial infarction, 17–21
overdrive, 116, 174
paradigms of, 185–186
premature ventricular contraction in,
    81f, 82–83
rate-modulated, 103–109 (*See also*
    Rate-modulated pacing)
rate of (*See* Rate)
safety, 43–44, 177

syncope in, 14–17, 71
temporary applications of, 88–93
  esophageal, 92–93
  transcutaneous, 89–92, 89f, 90f
  transvenous, 88–89
underdrive, 178
unipolar, 43–44, 44f
Pacing spike
  intermittent or erratic prolongation of,
    154–155, 155f
  in pulse-width programmability, 62–63,
    63f
  in strength-duration curve, 52, 53f
Pacing system analyzer (PSA), 175
Patient follow-up, 143–164. *See also*
    Follow-up, of pacemaker patient
Patient manipulation, of pacemaker, 158
Pectoral muscle stimulation, 157
Pediatric patients, 163
Peel-away sheath, 130f
pH measurement, in rate-modulated
    pacing, 108
Phantom programming, 175
Physical exam, follow-up, 143, 144t
Physiologic stress, rate-modulated pacing
    for, 103
Piezoelectrode, 103
Polarization resistance, 47–48, 48f, 175
Polyurethane, 175
Postventricular atrial refractory period
    (PVARP), 79, 79f, 175
  in DVI mode, 83
Power sources. *See also* Battery
  of permanent pacemaker, 28–31
  of temporary pacemaker, 42
Premature ventricular contraction
  in AV sequential pacing, 81f, 82–83
  crosstalk in, 95–96, 96f
  ECG of, 189
Programmability, 61–73, 176
  in dual-chamber pacing, 99–100, 100t
  external methods of, 61
  hysteresis, 70–71, 71f
  mode, 71–72
  noise-sensing circuit in, 66–67
  pulse-width, 62–64, 63f, 64f, 64t
  rate, 61–62, 62t
  refractory period, 68–69, 68f–70f, 70t

Programmability (*cont.*)
    sensitivity circuit and, 65–66, 67f, 68f
    of temporary pacemakers, 72–73, 72f,
        73f
    voltage, 65, 65f, 66t
Programming, phantom, 175
PSA (pacing system analyzer), 175
Pseudofusion beat, 176
Pseudomalfunction, 153, 154, 176
Pseudopseudofusion beat, 176
Pulse-width, 176
    programmability of, 62–64, 63f, 64f,
        64t

Q
QRS
    of atrioventricular node block, 4–6, 4f
    catecholamines on, 105–106, 106f
    of His bundle electrogram, 3, 3f
    nonsensing of, 155–156, 155f
    sensing of, 55–56, 56f
    sensitivity circuit on, 65–66, 67f, 68f
    in transcutaneous pacing, 91, 91f
    of unipolar *vs.* bipolar pacemaker, 41

R
R wave, 146–147
Radiation therapy, 161
Ramp pacing, 116, 117f
Rate
    change of, in ECG abnormality, 154
    maximum tracking rate, 80
    in permanent pacemakers,
        programmability of, 61–62, 62t
    in temporary pacemakers,
        programmability of, 72, 72f
    upper limit, in dual-chamber pacing,
        98–99
    upper rate limit, 80
Rate-modulated pacing, 103–109
    accelerometer motion sensor in,
        104–105
    catecholamines in, 105–106, 106f
    central oxygen saturation in, 108
    combined sensor utilization in, 108
    minute ventilation (respiration) in, 107,
        107f
    pH measurement in, 108

    rate-response algorithm in, 104f,
        108–109
    right ventricular pressure in, 106
    right ventricular stroke volume in, 106,
        106f
    temperature in, 105
    temporary, 109
    vibration sensor in, 103–104
Rate modulation, 176
Rate-responsive AV delay, 99, 176
Rate smoothing, 80, 108–109, 176
Reconfirmation ICD, 176
Reed switch, 176
    in external programming, 61
Refractory period, 177
    postventricular atrial, 79, 79f
    programmability of, 68–69, 68f–70f,
        70t
Resistance, 27, 177
    in polarization resistance, 47–48, 48f
Respiration, in rate-modulated pacing,
        107, 107f
Retrograde AV conduction, 177
Rheobase, 177
Rhythm, underlying, establishment of,
        146
Right ventricular pressure, in rate-
        modulated pacing, 106
Right ventricular stroke volume, in rate-
        modulated pacing, 106, 106f
Runaway pacemaker, 158–159

S
SA node conduction time, 10
Safety issues, in temporary pacemakers,
        43–44
Safety pacing, 177
Salt intake, for neurogenic syncope, 16–17
Scanning, 116, 117f
Scopolamine, 17
Seldinger technique, 129, 130f
Self-discharge rate, 29
Semiconductor, 32, 32f, 177
Sensing, 177
    inappropriate, 154, 155, 155f
    in pacing, 55–58, 56f–58f
Sensing threshold, 177
    evaluation of, 146–147, 148t

Sensitivity, in temporary pacemakers
  programming of, 73, 73f
  transvenous pacing with, 88
Sensitivity circuit, programmability of,
  65–66, 67f, 68f
Sensitivity value, 147
Sensor evaluation, 149
Sick sinus syndrome, 8–10
Silent atria, 78
Silicone, 177
Single-chamber pacemaker, 78
  transvenous temporary pacing with,
  88–89
Sinus node, overdrive suppression of, 9
Slew rate, 56, 58, 58f, 178
Smoothing, of rate, 80, 108–109, 176
Source impedance, 55–56, 178
Spike, 178
Stenosis, in hypertrophic obstructive
  cardiomyopathy, 12–13
Stimulus artifact amplitude, 41
Strength-duration curve, 52, 53f, 178
Stroke volume, in rate-modulated pacing,
  106, 106f
Subclavian stick technique, 130f
Subclavian vein, 128f, 138, 139f
Surgery, cardiac, temporary pacing after,
  140–141
Symptomatic bradycardia, 1
Syncope
  diagnostic clues in, 14–16, 15f
  hysteresis in, 71
  treatment in, 16–17
System impedance, 53

T
T-shock, 178
T wave, sensing of, 69, 70f
Tachy-brady syndrome, 9
Tachycardia. *See also* Antitachycardia
    therapy
  atrioventricular synchrony on, 86, 87f, 88
  detection of, implantable cardioverter
    defibrillator for, 115
  pacemaker-mediated, 96–98, 97f
  tachy-brady syndrome, 9
  temporary pacemaker therapy for,
    21–22

Telemetry, 178
  in hospital, 160–161
Temperature, in rate-modulated pacing,
    105
Threshold, 178
  acute, 167
  changes in, 53–54, 54f, 55f
  chronic, 169
  defibrillation, 171
  determination of, 51–53, 52t, 53f
  poor, in lack of capture, 152
Thrombosis, 158
Tilt, 178
  in constant voltage pacing, 49
Tilt test, 15–16, 15f
Timing cycles (intervals), in dual-chamber
    pacing, 78–80, 79f
Total atrial refractory period (TARP), 80,
    178
  on upper rate limit, 98–99
Transcutaneous electronic nerve
    stimulation (TENS), 121
Transcutaneous temporary pacing, 89–92,
    89f, 90f
Transtelephonic monitoring, 150, 151f,
    152f
Transvenous implantation
  permanent, 127–129, 128f
  temporary, 137–140, 138f, 139f, 140f
Transvenous pacing, 37–38, 38f
  temporary, 88–89
Transxiphoid approach, 132f
Trendelenburg position, 138–139
Triggered mode, 178

U
Underdrive pacing, 178
Unipolar, 179
  temporary pacing circuit of, 43–44, 44f
  vs. bipolar pacemaker, 37–41, 37f–39f
Upper rate limit, 80
  in DDD mode, 84
  in dual-chamber pacing, 98–99

V
VA interval, 80
Vagotonia, 5
Vasodepressor carotid hypertension, 12

Vasodepressor syncope, 15–16
VDD mode, 81–82, 81f–82f, 85t
VDI mode, 82–83, 85t
Ventilation, in rate-modulated pacing, 107,
   107f
Ventricular beat, premature, 81f, 82–83
   crosstalk in, 95–96, 96f
Ventricular pressure, in rate-modulated
   pacing, 106
Ventricular rate, smoothing of, 80
Ventricular refractory period (VRP),
   80
Ventricular safety pacing, 95–96
Ventricular tachycardia
   ICD for, 116
   temporary pacemaker therapy for,
     21–22
Verapamil, for pacemaker-mediated
   tachycardia, 97
Vibration sensor, in rate-modulated
   pacing, 103–104

Volt, 27, 179
Voltage
   and current threshold, 51–52, 52t
   programmability of, 65, 65f, 66t
   threshold, of unipolar *vs.* bipolar
     pacemaker, 40
VVI mode, 88
   ECG of, 187

W
Watt, 28, 179
Wenckebach phenomenon, 2, 179
   in rate-response algorithm, 109
   upper rate limit in, 98–99

X
Xylocaine (lidocaine), for esophageal
   catheter, 93

Z
Zinc mercuric oxide battery, 31